Critical Thinking
in the
Emergency Department

Skills to Assess, Analyze, and Act

Shelley Cohen, RN, BS, CEN

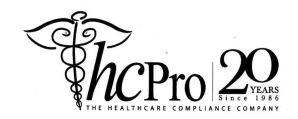

Critical Thinking in the Emergency Department: Skills to Assess, Analyze, and Act
by Shelley Cohen, RN, BS, CEN

Published by HCPro, Inc. Copyright ©2006 HCPro, Inc.

All rights reserved. Printed in the United States of America.   5   4   3   2   1

ISBN 1-57839-859-2

HCPro, Inc., provides information resources for the healthcare industry.

HCPro, Inc., is not affiliated in any way with the Joint Commission on Accreditation of Healthcare Organizations, which owns the JCAHO trademark.

Shelley Cohen, RN, BS, CEN, Author
Polly Gerber Zimmermann, RN, MS, MBA, CEN, Contributing Author
Rebecca Hendren, Managing Editor
Emily Sheahan, Group Publisher
Patrick Campagnone, Cover Designer
Mike Mirabello, Senior Graphic Artist
Jerrie Hildebrand, Layout Artist
Jean St. Pierre, Director of Operations
Darren Kelly, Production Coordinator
Matthew Kuhrt, Copyeditor
Sada Preisch, Proofreader

Advice given is general. Readers should consult professional counsel for specific legal, ethical, or clinical questions.

Arrangements can be made for quantity discounts. For more information, contact:

HCPro, Inc.
200 Hoods Lane
P.O. Box 1168
Marblehead, MA 01945
Telephone: 800/650-6787 or 781/639-1872
Fax: 781/639-2982
E-mail: *customerservice@hcpro.com*

Visit HCPro, Inc., at its World Wide Web sites: *www.hcpro.com* and *www.hcmarketplace.com*

09/2006
20972

Contents

Contents

Contents

List of figures

List of figures

Chapter 9

About the authors

Shelley Cohen, RN, BS, CEN

Shelley Cohen, RN, BS, CEN, is the founder and president of Health Resources Unlimited, a Tennessee-based healthcare education and consulting company (*www.hru.net*). Through her seminars for nursing professionals, Cohen coaches and educates healthcare workers and leaders across the country to provide the very best in patient care. She frequently presents her work on leadership and triage at national conferences.

When she is not speaking or teaching, Cohen works as a staff emergency department nurse and develops educational plans for a local emergency department, including strategies for new-graduate orientation. She also writes her monthly electronic publications—*Manager Tip of the Month* and *Triage Tip of the Month*—read by thousands of professionals across the United States.

She is an editorial advisor for *Strategies for Nurse Managers*, published by HCPro, Inc., and is a frequent contributor to *Nursing Management* magazine. She co-authored the book *A Practical Guide to Recruitment and Retention: Skills for Nurse Managers*, published by HCPro, Inc.

She has a background in emergency, critical care, and occupational medicine. Over the past 30 years, she has worked both as a staff nurse and nurse executive.

When her laptop computer shuts down and her stethoscope comes off, Cohen puts on her child-advocacy hat and, with the help of her husband, Dennis, provides foster care to area children.

Contributing author: Polly Gerber Zimmermann, RN, MS, MBA, CEN

Polly Gerber Zimmermann, RN, MS, MBA, CEN, has been in active in emergency and medical-surgical nursing clinical practice for more than 29 years and involved in nurse educating for more than 10 years. She was the senior course manager for the nursing division of the National Center for Advanced Medical Education, and is a tenured assistant professor in the Department of Nursing at the Harry S. Truman College (Chicago). Under her guidance, the school's curriculum instituted an integration of prioritization principles and critical thinking that resulted in the school's students improving from below to above national average results in these areas on standardized test scores.

Zimmermann is a frequent national speaker and has published more than 200 times. In addition, she writes test items that score high in critical thinking for national standardized tests, including HESI, NLN, NCLEX, and Excelsior College (Regents).

She was an associate editor and section editor of the Managers Forum for the *Journal of Emergency Nursing* for more than 10 years and is a contributing editor; section editor for the emergency section of the *American Journal of Nursing*. She has also been a legal expert/consultant in more than 45 cases.

Critical thinking in the emergency department

LEARNING OBJECTIVE

After reading this section, the participant should be able to

- describe the characteristics of the emergency department that require good decision-making skills

Back to basics

After being an emergency department (ED) nurse for quite awhile, you get to know how other ED nurses think. Your first thought may just be to flip directly to the tools and forms in this book—but don't go there yet.

To be successful at mentoring and supporting critical thinking, you need to be willing to learn the basic principles behind critical thinking. These fundamental concepts are generic for all nurses, regardless of the specialty they are working in.

To make the most of this book as your resource for critical thinking, consider making time to review all of the content before you implement the helpful tools. It may be tempting to just start using them immediately, but you would not expect a new nurse to understand the relationship between blood loss and delay in blood pressure changes without some foundational knowledge of anatomy and physiology. That same principle applies here. The tools are not the answer: the answer lies in grasping the concepts of critical thinking.

Critical thinking and the ED setting

The emergency department is a place of "unknowns," which requires nursing staff to display unique qualities and high levels of critical thinking, both as individuals and as part of a team.

The unknowns that make the ED such an interesting place include the following:

- How many patients will arrive?
- When they will arrive?
- How many will be high acuity or low acuity?
- How many will require immediate life-saving measures?
- How many have the potential for violence?
- How long will those requiring admission need to wait for their inpatient bed?
- How many will require transfer to a higher-skill-level facility?

The constantly changing, sometimes chaotic environment is what drives some nurses to this specialty. The team whose members get to know one another's strengths and weaknesses quickly demonstrates good decision-making skills. A sense of unspoken trust usually develops among not only the nursing team, but also the medical providers. In this environment of rapidly changing, multiple-patient assignments and constant sorting (triage), the ED nurse needs to have all the attributes of a critical thinker, and needs to know how to use strategies that aid critical thinking.

Emergency department nurses will be faced with patients who present through a variety of points of entry and exit, and with an unlimited number of problems and needs. ED nurses must be able to make decisions that apply to a multitude of scenarios for every age-specific patient category.

The three main areas in which the ED nurse will apply critical thinking skills are triage, treatment, and disposition.

Triage

Whether patients present via the Emergency Medical Services (EMS) system or independently, a sorting process, called triage, occurs to determine their potential for demise, so those most in need of care are seen first.

This area of nursing practice requires not only critical thinking, but also experience. The most successful triage nurses are those who possess a combination of these two elements and can apply them for effective decision-making. Clearly, this is not a process new graduate nurses are prepared for without extensive training and ED work experience.

Attributes of critical thinking during triage

The following examples demonstrate application of the concepts and approaches of critical thinking at this entry point of ED care. Strategies and attributes of critical thinking during the triage process include the following abilities:

Independent thinker

- Identifies and initiates appropriate standing orders.

- Recognizes when patient volume will require more support at triage and notifies the charge nurse before long delays occur for triage.

Evaluates evidence and facts

- At triage, a patient states he was not trying to kill himself. The police officer who presents with the patient shows the nurse a note and weapon found at the scene.

Explores consequences before making decisions or taking action

- Although the department exam areas are full of patients, the triage nurse realizes that the patient presenting from the county jail with a police officer should not be held waiting in the triage area.

Evaluates policy

- Recognizes that although the visitor is demanding to see the patient now, the patient's tracking board displays a security icon. The charge nurse is contacted prior to allowing any visitors through the door.

Confident in decisions

- A provider challenges the triage nurse about a decision the nurse made at triage. The nurse refers the provider to the written protocols that were followed to come to the decision.

Asks pertinent questions

- Understands that no assumptions should be made at triage. Every patient presenting is asked, "Have you had an injury?"

- Asks parent what dose of fever medicine the child was given.

Displays curiosity

- At end of shift, checks on status of patients who were a challenge at triage. Reviews patient outcomes and determines if the triage process or decision was appropriate.

Rejects incorrect information

- Despite the fact that the caregiver claims the child is eating and drinking, the triage nurse notes the child has dry mucous membranes and produces no tears when crying.

Treatment

The treatment area of the ED brings its own set of challenges with multiple patient assignments and varying levels of patient acuity. This rapid turnover environment presents the critical thinker with the opportunity to demonstrate the ability to make decisions in a fast-paced setting. During this point of care, nurses are more involved as a team of critical thinkers working together, contributing decision-making comments that lead to improved patient outcomes. Typically, a nurse serves in the role of charge or team leader to ensure the merging of patient flow and staff resources. Collaborative relationships and efforts with the medical staff of the ED provide opportunities for nurses to gain clinical knowledge that reflects their ability to make good decisions.

Attributes of critical thinking during treatment

Strategies and attributes of critical thinking during the triage process include the following abilities:

Independent thinker

- Rationalizes which patient needs attention next.
- Recognizes the need to call pharmacy to ensure two medications are compatible.

Evaluates evidence and facts

- Notes critical lab values, reassesses patient, and approaches provider with information and request for orders.

Explores consequences before making decisions or taking action

- Patient's family is requesting fluids/food for a patient who is being evaluated for mental status change. Knowing that patients who may require surgery should be NPO, reviews head CT results and notes they are normal without sign of subdural or lesion.

Evaluates policy

- Patient requests that the police not be notified of the assault from his or her spouse. Nurse refers to hospital policy requiring that all assaults be reported and offers patient safety options prior to discharge.

Confident in decisions

- During a resuscitative effort, a physician orders a dose of medication that is twice the dose recommended by the American Heart Association. Despite the urgent needs of the patient, the nurse reads the order back to the physician and questions the dose.

Asks pertinent questions

- The nurse is comfortable saying, "This patient is concerning me as she may be an atypical presentation. How do you feel about my doing an EKG on her?"

Displays curiosity

- When caring for an asthma patient, the nurse approaches the provider and, while updating him or her on the patient's status, inquires, "Do you know anything about asthma patients being given magnesium in the ED? I read about this last week but have never seen it given for asthma before. What do you think?"

Rejects incorrect information

- When reviewing laboratory results, notes a patient has dangerously low blood sugar. After reevaluating the patient, the nurse performs a finger-stick glucose test and finds the patient to have normal-range blood sugar. Upon discussion with the lab, it is determined there is an inpatient with the same first and last name of this ED patient.

Disposition

After receiving treatment, the options for where a patient goes next include

- discharge home
- return/admitted to nursing home as resident
- referred to dentist or doctor's office
- transferred to another facility
- sent to the morgue
- admitted to the hospital
- discharge to law enforcement officials

With more patients waiting for an empty exam room, there is always a push to move patients out of the department as efficiently as we can. Nurses feel pressure as they try to ensure all the discharge/admission/transfer criteria are met for each patient. This is an additional obstacle for nurses trying to employ critical thinking as they disposition patients. With so many risk-management and follow-up details to consider, nurses may at times forget some details due to this pressure.

As part of the disposition process, nurses need to consider the following:

- Reevaluate vital signs, pain status, neurological status
- Review documentation to ensure completeness and thoroughness
- Patients with limited English proficiency take longer to disposition
- Some discharge instructions are lengthy
- Time to await appropriate person, other than patient, to review disposition information
- Admissions being held in the department that require ongoing nursing assessments

We expect a great deal in a short period of time from ED nurses at the point of disposition. Make sure they have the time and resources they need to accomplish everything with critical thinking and critical documenting.

Attributes of critical thinking during disposition

Strategies and attributes of critical thinking during the disposition process include the following abilities:

Independent thinker

- Recognizes the discharge orders from the provider are premature and the patient will need to wait for an evaluation by the mental health worker.

Evaluates evidence and facts

- Although patient claims, "I can handle this by myself," nurse notes patient is unable to demonstrate safe use of crutches. Suggests to provider that the patient be given a walker.

Explores consequences before making decisions or taking action

- Asks who will be driving the patient home from the ED prior to administering a narcotic for pain management.

Confident in decisions

- Although a particular dressing is ordered for the patient's burn, the nurse recognizes the fragile skin of the elderly patient and suggests another option that will not require tape on the patient's skin.

Asks pertinent questions

- Asks elderly patient who lives alone, "Is there someone who can help you with these dressing changes when you get home?"

Displays curiosity

- While holding a patient being admitted for Guillain-Barre Syndrome, the nurse asks the provider about what clues led him or her to this diagnosis.

Listens to others and is able to give feedback

- Makes sure the new parents understand the discharge instructions for their eight-day-old newborn by asking them to repeat them back. The ED nurse has the parents demonstrate the correct method of taking a rectal temperature.

Encouraging the development of critical thinking in ED nurses

Much of critical thinking needed in the ED setting does come from work experiences and particular patient scenarios that nurses tend to "bookmark" in their minds. All ED nurses should be actively involved in the orientation and development of both new graduate nurses and experienced nurses who join the ED setting. Without passing along these bookmarked events, we cannot help others to develop their critical thinking capabilities.

We want ED nurses who are able to

- recognize a problem
- know what to do
- know when to do it
- know how to do it
- know why they are doing it

ED nurses know what outcomes they want for each patient and recognize how they affect these outcomes. Recognizing the role critical thinking plays in achieving these desired outcomes is the first step to creating and achieving an environment that promotes sound judgments.

To promote critical thinking in the ED, incorporate the ENA's *Code of Ethics for Emergency Nurses* in the process of ongoing development by having all staff sign a commitment to this ethical practice. Let nursing staff know what is expected from them regarding their abilities in decision-making and then promote and encourage their ongoing development.

It is a privilege to be an ED nurse and be at the side of a patient and family when they are in unexpected need of medical care. It takes a special person to be an ED nurse and with that comes a tremendous responsibility and power to make the best decisions for the patients entrusting their care to us.

Defining critical thinking

By Polly Gerber Zimmermann, RN, MS, MBA, CEN

LEARNING OBJECTIVE

After reading this section, the participant should be able to

- identify the key aspects of critical thinking and how nurses develop competency

Why critical thinking?

For educators and nurse leaders, critical thinking is like the weather: Everybody is talking about it, but nobody seems to know what to do about it. Passing the NCLEX only validates that new graduates have the *minimal* amount of knowledge needed to provide safe nursing care. Application of clinical critical thinking and judgment is at the heart of what makes a healthcare provider *nurse* (as a verb) compared to being a technician who completes tasks by rote. Critical thinking is at the core of safe nursing practice, and thus encouraging its development in every nurse should be an aim for all educators.

Becoming a professional nurse

Nursing is a hands-on profession for which clinical experience plays a crucial role in professional development. Nurses have to progress through various levels before they reach proficiency. Managers and educators need to appreciate that new graduate nurses are at a different level, with different needs, than experienced nurses in their professional critical thinking.

Benner's stages of growth

Benner (1984) is well known for identifying and describing the five stages through which nurses proceed in their professional growth. Benner's stages are

Beginner: Has little experience and skills, learning by rote, completing education requirements.

Advanced beginner: Can perform adequately with some judgment, usually at this stage upon graduation.

Competent: Able to foresee long-range goals and are mastering skills. Still lack the experience to make instantaneous decisions based on intuition. Most nurses take up to one year to reach this stage.

Proficient: View situation as a whole, rather than its parts. Able to develop a solution.

Expert: Intuition and decision-making are instantaneous. Most nurses take at least five years in an area of practice to reach this stage.

So how do you take your inexperienced graduates and set them on the road to proficiency? And how do you help your more experienced nurses—who may have been practicing for years, yet you would never label them experts—reach that higher level? This book provides information, strategies, and tools to help you coach nurses at all stages of development as they hone their critical thinking skills, improve their judgment, and become better nurses. Chapter 3 discusses teaching critical thinking in a classroom setting, and other chapters include ongoing strategies for developing critical thinking in the clinical environment.

The goal in encouraging and developing critical thinking is to help nurses progress effectively through the stages of development. No one wants 10-year nurse employees who have the equivalent of one year of experience simply repeated 10 times.

So what is critical thinking?

Alfaro-LeFevre (1999) defines critical thinking as careful, deliberate, outcome-focused (results-oriented) thinking that is mastered for a context. Critical thinking is based on scientific method; the nursing process; a high level of knowledge, skills, and experience; professional standards; a positive attitude toward learning; and a code of ethics. It includes elements of constant reevaluation, self-correction, and continual striving for improvement.

Some of the characteristics of people who display critical thinking include open-mindedness, the ability to see things from more than one perspective, awareness of one's own strengths and weaknesses, and ongoing striving for improvement. The strategies commonly (and often subconsciously) used in critical thinking include reasoning (inductive reasoning, such as specific to general, or deductive reasoning, such as general to specific), pattern recognition, repetitive hypothesizing, mental representation, and intuition.

In the practical world of clinical nursing, critical thinking is the ability of nurses to see patients' needs uniquely and respond appropriately, beyond or in spite of the orders. The ability to think critically is developed through ongoing knowledge gathering, experience, reading the literature, and continuous quality improvement by reviewing one's own patient charts. An example of a nurse who displays critical thinking is when a physician orders acetaminophen (Tylenol) for a patient's fever, and the nurse questions the order because the patient has hepatitis C. A critical thinker goes beyond being a "robo-nurse" who simply does as he or she is told.

In Croskerry's study (2003), 32 types of misperceptions and biases (cognitive disposition to respond) were identified in clinical decision-making. Everyone is influenced by what they see most often, most recently, or most dramatically. Cognitive errors may be avoided by always striving to consider alternatives; by decreasing reliance on memory (instead, use cognitive aids such as reference books); by using cognitive forcing strategies, such as a protocol; by taking time to think; and by having rapid and reliable feedback and follow-up to avoid repeating errors.

The overarching goal is to help shorten new graduate nurses' on-the-job learning curve, and give directed assistance to all nurses in their critical thinking development.

Del Bueno's definition of critical thinking

There are many definitions of critical thinking, and one of the most helpful is Dorothy Del Bueno's Performance-Based Development System. Del Bueno determined that nursing competency involves three skills: interpersonal skills, technical skills, and critical thinking.

Del Bueno defines critical thinking in a clinical setting with the following four aspects:

- Can the nurse recognize the patient's problem?
- Can the nurse safely and effectively manage the problem?
- Does the nurse have a relative sense of urgency?
- Does the nurse do the right thing for the right reason?

Del Bueno discussed an example from her work on responses to a taped scenario of a one-day postop trauma patient. On the tape shown to nurses, the patient suddenly becomes diaphoretic, pale, short of breath with tachypnea, and holds the right side of the chest, complaining of pain. An ABG result is given showing respiratory alkalosis. The expectation is that nurses will recognize this is a potential pulmonary embolism or pneumothorax (an alteration in respiration), manage the patient with oxygen, assess breath sounds, raise the head of the bed, call the physician, etc. And experienced nurses should anticipate physician orders, such as a portable chest x-ray or an EKG. But Del Bueno found that 75% of inexperienced and 25% of experienced nurses said they would manage the patient's alkalosis by *only* having the patient breathe into a paper bag.

Overall, she found that only 25%–30% of inexperienced nurses (less than one year of clinical experience) had acceptable results. The range of acceptable results was from 12% to 60%, and there was no difference between nurses' performance based on their educational preparation and/or whether they had previous healthcare experience (such as being a technician or an LPN). She found that 65% of experienced nurses had acceptable results, and that the number was higher (85%) in some specialties. Overall, she found that nurses' greatest limitations were in recognition and management of renal and neurological problems.

References

Alfaro-LeFevre, R. 1999. *Critical Thinking in Nursing: A Practical Approach.* Philadelphia: WB Saunders.

Benner P. 1984. *From Novice to Expert.* Menlo Park, CA: Addison-Wesley.

Brown, S. 2000. "Shock of the new." *Nursing Times* 96 (38): 27.

Charnley, E. 1999. "Occupational stress in the newly qualified staff nurse." *Nursing Standard* 13 (29): 32–37.

Croskerry, P. 2003. "The importance of cognitive errors in diagnosis and strategies to minimize them." *Academy of Medicine* 78 (8): 775–780.

Del Bueno, D. 2001. "Buyer beware: The cost of competence." *Nursing Economics* 19 (6): 259–257.

Gries, M. 2000. "Don't leave grads lost at sea." *Nursing Spectrum.* Accessed on July 27, 2006 from *http://community.nursingspectrum.com/MagazineArticles/article.cfm?AID=800.*

Huber, D. 2000. *Leadership and Nursing Care Management,* 2nd ed. Philadelphia: WB Saunders.

Norris, T. L. 2005. "Making the transition from student to professional nurse." In B. Cherry and S. R. Jacob, *Contemporary Nursing: Issues, Trends, & Management,* 3rd ed. St. Louis: Elsevier/Mosby.

Tingle, C. A. 2000. "Workplace advocacy as a transition tool." *LSNA Insider.* June.

Zimmermann, P. G. 2002. "Guiding principles at triage: Advice for new triage nurses." *Journal of Emergency Nursing* 28 (1): 24–33.

Zimmerman, P. G., and R. D. Herr. 2006. *Triage Nursing Secrets.* St. Louis: Elsevier/Mosby.

New graduate nurses and critical thinking

By Polly Gerber Zimmermann, RN, MS, MBA, CEN

LEARNING OBJECTIVE

After reading this section, the participant should be able to

- analyze the factors that contribute to new graduates' lack of critical thinking and strategies to counteract this

Why don't new graduates think critically?

Educators' and nurse leaders' desire to develop nurses' critical thinking is undoubtedly more pressing for new graduate nurses. You may wonder why these nurses, who have just completed their education, do not display the qualities and skills you either expect or want. It's important to understand that new graduates face many stresses as they transition from students to registered nurses, and these stresses impede their ability to learn and progress.

Stresses for new graduate nurses

Charnley (1999) identified four categories that lead to stress in novice nurses:

1. **Reality of practice:** They think they are supposed to have all the answers, are overwhelmed by the volume of work, and feel guilty because they cannot spend more time with patients.

2. **Unfamiliarity with the structure of the organization:** They spend valuable time looking for supplies.

3. **Lack of professional relationships:** They lack an understanding of the roles of healthcare providers, and their dependence on other staff may cause anxiety. They often lack mentors and support people.

4. **Lack of clinical judgment:** They have decreased confidence in their skills and decision-making abilities. This leads to apprehension.

Other special needs of new graduates have been identified, including the following (Brown, 2000; Charnley, 1999; Gries, 2000; Huber, 2000; Tingle, 2000):

Interpersonal skills/communication: They struggle with interactions with other providers in making rounds, clarifying orders, and interdisciplinary team conferences. They may miss some communication or instruction from an experienced nurse because they don't understand what the routine or slang involves. For example, one unit may refer to a septic workup as "culturing every hole." The new graduate does not understand that this standard order set includes blood cultures x2, sputum culture, urine culture, and stool culture.

Clinical: Though new nurses possess the clinical knowledge, they lack the experience that increases effectiveness, efficiency, and correctness.

Organization: This includes organization of skills and the day, often exacerbated by feeling overwhelmed and unsure how to prioritize.

Delegation: New nurses often feel uncomfortable delegating to more experienced and/or older assistants. This is exacerbated by a lack of leadership skills and trust/personal knowledge of the assistants.

Priority setting: Initially, there is a tendency to focus on tasks, rather than critical thinking planning.

Assertiveness: There can be hesitancy to say no or to understand the difference between being assertive and being aggressive.

As outlined above, the transition into practice includes a lot of stress. But new graduates can be helped to overcome the stressors and grow in critical thinking more easily when the orientation process recognizes and deals with these stresses.

Strategies to minimize stress

There are aspects you can add to orientation and for ongoing use that will minimize these stressors for new graduates. Possibilities include:

- Holding regular support group meetings with fellow orientees.

- Using a mentor or assigning a buddy (or sponsor) who builds a relationship and will follow the nurse for at least a year.

- Holding a treasure hunt for supplies or other departments during their first week of work. It will help their confidence if they know where the laboratory is located when someone stops them in the hall to ask.

- Holding a roundtable of the institution's staff nurses who have been out of school for two to five years, who can offer tips and support. (These nurses will be experienced enough to have learned, but not so experienced to have forgotten.)

- Spending a day rounding with a teaching physician who frequently admits to the unit.

- Emphasizing the importance of just "tell somebody" when something is abnormal, even if they do not know the cause or the solution. Alerting someone else will help new nurses learn. Make clear that waiting, assessing, and hoping is not a good solution.

New graduates' levels of development

When learning a new field, there are four classic stages through which the person proceeds:

- Unconsciously incompetent
- Consciously incompetent
- Consciously competent
- Unconsciously competent

The most dangerous situation is when nurses do not realize what they do not know. The best orientee is the one who realizes when to ask for help. Surprisingly, weaker students are frequently very confident, in part because they don't grasp how much there is to learn or the potential risks.

A contributing factor to this phenomenon is that newer nurses are often placed on the off shifts with other inexperienced nurses. This can limit their exposure to more-experienced nurses and they do not realize their deficiencies since their coworkers have similar levels of knowledge and judgment.

Part of developing critical thinking and orientees' ongoing self-knowledge should include encouraging them to think about "In what areas do I still need to grow?" Keep the issue of critical thinking and anticipation of potential patient complications in the forefront.

Prioritization

Prioritization typically is one of the most difficult aspects for new nurses to learn. They know if something is "normal" or "not normal," but struggle to know how much importance to attach to these classifications. Many educators and managers think new graduates will automatically pick up this discernment, but this often does not happen until after considerable time, exposure, and experience.

New graduates struggle to prioritize the needs within one patient, within a team of patients, and/or between patient and administration needs. It is necessary to provide rules and principles they can use until they develop and internalize their own clinical judgment and instinct.

Prioritization principles: Assessment

Many of the following concepts may seem simplistic and obvious, but remember that experienced nurses often forget what they, as new graduates, didn't know. Discuss the following aspects in a critical-thinking class, and include them during orientation and throughout new graduates' initial development:

Review Maslow's Hierarchy of Needs and ABCD: While familiar content, many new graduates have not specifically identified that "D for disability" includes mental status / level of consciousness (LOC), neurological and motor function, and pain. Pain, while not a good thing, is not always the worst thing. Sometimes in an effort to overcompensate for the past when analgesia received inadequate attention, pain is given almost absolute priority in the nursing curriculum.

Two common areas of weakness in new graduates are failure to ask all aspects of a pain assessment (PQRST) and failure to note the severity within the ABCD prioritization. Use examples where the type of pain and/or location, rather than severity, alerts the nurse to the problem, such as a substernal pressure that the patient rates as a 5. Use examples in which the severity matters: a significant shock (Circulation) takes priority over a mild wheezing (Breathing).

Onset (sudden over gradual): True sudden onset of symptoms can signal a catastrophic event. It is a true "sudden" onset if the patient can recall the exact time or activity when it began, and the maximum intensity is reached immediately (in less than one minute).

Actual over potential: A common error of new graduates is to focus on a "more important" potential future problem than what is currently going on. For instance, they assume the asthmatic patient who states he or she will stop his or her prednisone will take priority over someone who is currently experiencing low blood pressure. Emphasize first things first: Treat actual problems before preventing a future one.

Systemic over local (life before limb): Something that has a systemic implication, or involves multiple systems, is a priority. If no other access can be obtained, an IV is started in the leg to administer the medication to stop continuous statis epilepticus.

Trends: A trend, as opposed to an isolated incident, could be an indication of something more serious. Trends include a steady progressive decline, minor symptoms that recur repeatedly or increase in severity, and/or symptoms that are associated with other definitive (especially systemic) changes.

Compared to the patient's normal: Recognition of the same significant symptoms ("This is like the last time I had a kidney stone") or identification of a new distinction ("This is different from any other headache I had before") is important. When the complaint is "ordinary," such as a headache, remember there must be a reason why the patient thought it was important enough to report. Always consider the caregivers' perception of changes in the patient, as they know the person better than anyone.

For example, one geriatric patient was reassured by three nurses that her reported urinary incontinence was "typical" for the elderly. It took the fourth nurse to assess this symptom as a new onset, with urinary burning, and take the necessary actions to diagnose the patient's new urinary tract infection.

Patient demographics: Certain groups are more vulnerable for rapid worsening or atypical symptoms and should receive more consideration. This includes the immunosuppressed, whether by age (the very young and the very old), medication (steroid administration), disease (diabetes mellitus, HIV/AIDS), or past history (splenectomy, donor organ recipient). Similarly, greater concern should be given to patients with multiple comorbidities (their systems are already taxed for coping and will be more easily overwhelmed), or a history of the "worst-case scenario" in the past for these symptoms (e.g., "This is just like I felt when I had my heart attack").

Prioritization principles: Time management

Medications tend to be a priority and new graduates should be encouraged to consider the type and timing of medications. Anti-diabetic medications and antibiotics are usually given priority because of the consequences if they are not given in a timely manner. If two antibiotics are ordered for the same time, give the one with the shortest interval until the next dose first.

In school, nursing assessment and teaching are emphasized. The reality is that most hospitalized patients have a "diagnosis" and one of nursing's main functions is to properly administer the treatments prescribed for the patient's improvement. Why is the patient here? Make sure the "cures" are being administered.

Prioritization principles: Administrative

Patients before paperwork: Students from a heavily regulated industry, such as licensed practical nurses who worked in long-term care facilities, or those who truly understand legal implications, tend to overemphasize the documentation. Remind them that "post" charting is allowed if identified as such.

Stop any harm immediately: Those inexperienced in leadership tend to focus on others dealing with problems rather than directly taking care of it themselves. If an aide is making an error, go in and correct it now rather than telling the charge nurse, asking for more inservices, writing up an incident report, or even speaking to the aide at the end of the shift.

WHAT rather than WHO: An inexperienced nurse is likely to be intimidated and respond first to an authority figure who is barking orders. A serious patient need is always first. Have them role-play stating, "I must take care of this first, then I can be back and talk with you in about a minute."

Remind learners when talking about prioritization that everyone does receive care even if they are not first. Prioritization just recognizes that one person can only do so much at a time and there are competing demands. Prioritization involves the right care to the right person at the right time for the right reason.

Identifying worst-case scenarios, stereotypes, and expected abnormal findings

Worst-case scenarios

Another significant area in which new graduates need help is identifying and ruling out the worst-case scenario that could happen with a complaint. People make decisions heavily influenced by what they experience most often, most recently, or most dramatically in relation to the current situation. New graduates have mainly been exposed to textbook stable cases in clinical experiences.

Give new graduates examples and specifically identify what would be the worst complication. Ask them how they would know the worst-case scenario was occurring when dealing with any patient, condition, or scenario. The one-day postoperative patient may be restless due to pain, but has shock been ruled out? How would you do that? This is particularly important to stress during a critical-thinking class, but it should also be brought up again and again. Remember, repetition is the mother of all learning. New graduates should know that for each patient they take care of, they should first think, "What is the worst-case scenario?" so that this may be ruled out as necessary, and the process should eventually become automatic.

There is a familiar phrase used in medicine, "When you hear hoofbeats, think horses, not zebras." It illustrates the overarching principle that nurses should first consider the most common causes for a patient's presentation, but be alert to the fact there are some "zebras" out there. Don't miss them.

Stereotypes

It can be helpful to include common misconceptions (which are often subconscious) in illustrations. For example, common stereotypes may include that psychiatric patients don't have physical problems, or that all old people are a little bit confused. Nurses should ascertain whether the elderly patient with new-onset confusion has low glucose, low pulse-oximeter reading, or a urinary tract infection. False assumptions can lead to a wrong action.

Expected abnormal findings

What is an expected finding for this given condition? Make the distinction that significant "abnormal" findings are not a concern when they are a part of that patient's known medical condition. It is not alarming that a patient with pneumonia admitted for intravenous antibiotics has an elevated white blood cell count (WBC). It is more necessary to know if the WBC is higher, lower, or the same since starting the antibiotics. Similarly, it is not alarming that the patient with pancreatitis has amylase and lipase levels three times the normal value—that is how the diagnosis is made. It is more important to rule out serious complications such as hypocalcemia, hypovolemia, hypoxia, or severe pain.

Ongoing development

Awareness is the first step toward beginning to change behavior. Orientation often focuses on "how we do things here," and includes forms, policies, and the mission statement.

Orientation also should include a purposeful identification and focus on critical thinking. Discussion should include making clinical correlations, applying them to each patient's unique presentation, understanding the reason things are being done, and focusing on the most essential aspects in the proper order. Bringing these types of approaches to the forefront will help the new graduate understand what is needed to succeed.

References

Alfaro-LeFevre, R. 1999. *Critical Thinking in Nursing: A Practical Approach*. Philadelphia: WB Saunders.

Benner, P. 1984. *From Novice to Expert*. Menlo Park, CA: Addison-Wesley.

Brown, S. 2000. "Shock of the new." *Nursing Times* 96 (38): 27.

Charnley, E. 1999. "Occupational stress in the newly qualified staff nurse." *Nursing Standard* 13 (29): 32–37.

Croskerry, P. 2003. "The importance of cognitive errors in diagnosis and strategies to minimize them." *Academy of Medicine* 78 (8): 775–780.

Del Bueno, D. 2001. "Buyer beware: The cost of competence." *Nursing Economics* 19 (6): 259–257.

Gries, M. 2000. "Don't leave grads lost at sea." *Nursing Spectrum*. Accessed on July 27, 2006 from *http://community.nursingspectrum.com/MagazineArticles/article.cfm?AID=800*.

Huber, D. 2000. *Leadership and Nursing Care Management*, 2nd ed. Philadelphia: WB Saunders.

Norris, T. L. 2005. "Making the transition from student to professional nurse." In B. Cherry and S. R. Jacob, *Contemporary Nursing: Issues, Trends, & Management*, 3rd ed. St. Louis: Elsevier/Mosby.

Tingle, C. A. 2000. "Workplace advocacy as a transition tool." *LSNA Insider* (June).

Zimmermann, P. G. 2002. "Guiding principles at triage: Advice for new triage nurses." *Journal of Emergency Nursing* 28 (1): 24–33.

Zimmerman, P. G. and R. D. Herr. 2006. *Triage Nursing Secrets*. St. Louis: Elsevier/Mosby.

Chapter 3

The critical thinking classroom

By Polly Gerber Zimmermann, RN, MS, MBA, CEN

LEARNING OBJECTIVE

After reading this section, the participant should be able to

- utilize the classroom environment to teach, promote, and support the development of critical thinking

Critical thinking can be taught

The tendency is to view critical thinking as an abstract formula to memorize. Rather, it is a process of applying acquired textbook knowledge to the clinical setting and specific patients. All nurses usually need some initial assistance in applying their knowledge to the situation, particularly for high-volume, high-risk, or infrequent patient presentations with which they have had little familiarity during their education or experience.

Classes that discuss and teach critical thinking can be beneficial for both new graduates and more experienced nurses. New graduates and new hires will benefit from classes held during orientation, but it also may be useful to periodically schedule general-attendance classes so that other nurses may participate.

Background preparation

Teacher preparation

Educators can tend to spend excessive energy on "what" to teach. Just as important is "how" to teach—determining the best way to communicate the information so learning takes place. When planning an educational session, focus less on "What am I going to say today?" and more on "What are my listeners going to learn today?"

Teaching is not pouring wisdom into passive listeners. The teacher is a guide for active participation through a learning experience. Watch the audience's responses. That is the only way to perceive the need to repeat material, vary the presentation, or illustrate the content's application for this group.

Consider the learner's motivation

Why will attendees be motivated to learn? The driving force for all ordinary behavior is "What's in it for me?" Avoid the "Field of Dreams" approach—i.e., if we plan it, they will come and learn. Instead, use the human tendency toward selfishness—what's in it for me?—to teaching's advantage. Further breaking down that number one motivation reveals the three main aspects people want from education sessions. People want to

- get something accomplished/meet their goals
- receive personal recognition, power, or influence
- have social interaction and enjoyment

Most of us are usually more influenced by one factor than another, but there are aspects of all three in everyone. Time spent in the classroom should meet all three purposes. Give certificates; have checklists to complete; give personal, positive, public praise; and add humor or games.

Generational differences

Understanding motivational aspects is important when considering today's multigenerational work force. Everyone is influenced by the time in which they were raised, when they developed their mindset, values, priorities, and styles. As the Arab proverb says, "People resemble their times more than they resemble their parents."

Baby Boomers are individuals born between 1946–1964. The average age for registered nurses is 44 to 47 years. Baby Boomers are more likely to act out of a sense of duty and a drive to accomplish.

Generation Xers are those born between 1965–1980. They want independence and flexibility; they want to know "Why?" (as they focus on results); and they want fun. If an activity is not worthwhile to them, they do not feel a sense of obligation to stick it out and will check out physically and/or mentally.

Generation Y is the generation born between 1981–2006. They are entering the workplace with high expectations for themselves, their employers, and their managers, and expect coaching, training, and support to help them achieve their goals.

Many educators fall into the Baby Boomer age category, whereas new graduate nurses often fall into the Generation X or Generation Y categories. Remember that approaches used for the established work force, or even for you when you were a new graduate, may not work now. It's important to tailor learning experiences to meet the needs of all generations in your classes.

Professional nurses' goals

David Shore (1997) defined what professionals want from their educational offerings: They want to be an ACE. Specifically, they expect *Access* (to peers, resources, and networking), *Credentialing* (external validation of what they know and whether it is still correct), and *Education* (information to make a demonstrable, practical difference in their practice).

Keep these expectations in mind when planning learning experiences. Also note that experienced nurses are very interested in regulations (e.g., "JCAHO requires . . . ") or legal requirements (e.g., "In this case, a nurse was sued for . . . ").

Setting the stage

Classroom environment

The classroom environment plays a key role in your critical-thinking course. Create an atmosphere that awakens the participant's whole brain and senses. Communicate, even on a subconscious level, that this is an enjoyable, desirable place and activity.

Seating: As much as possible, use a half-circle for small groups, and a fishbone configuration for larger groups. Avoid having a group at a table with stragglers in the row behind. Avoid hiders: participation is necessary for learning.

Use color: One study found that visual aids with color and symbols increased long-term retention by 14–38%.

Peripheral learning: We use sight for 75% of our learning. While we speak at 125 words per minute, we think at about 600 words per minute. Give the learner something to do with the extra 475-word capacity. When their mind or eyes start to drift, let them fall on educational posters.

If it is a dedicated classroom, make posters that specifically apply to the content that is being taught. If it is a generic classroom, use prevention and healthcare associations' free posters—then even the housekeeping staff learns.

Music: Play upbeat music before class, during breaks, and after class. Baroque is recommended because it matches the rhythm of the heart and enhances learning. Use lively pop music with a distinct beat you can dance to—it will pump up the energy in the room.

Frequent breaks: Experts recommend taking a five-minute "exercise" break every 40–50 minutes, but it's even more effective to take a one-minute break every 25 minutes or so. Set a kitchen timer and, when it dings, announce that it's time for a break and turn on the music. Encourage general arm stretching, walking around, etc. Indicate participation is optional.

After one minute, turn off the music and start class, usually with joke. These breaks should be in addition to the scheduled longer break midway through the class. Teachers fear these breaks will create a loss of control of the classroom but that does not happen with adults when done with purposeful actions and explanations. Many students indicate "the music break" was one of their favorite aspects of the class.

There are many reasons to take these frequent breaks. Necessary bathroom breaks are then quickly facilitated without disrupting the classroom—and those who straggle back in miss the reward of humor. Exercise increases cognitive functioning, attention, and alertness. It pulls in the kinesthetic learners and individuals who have minor attention-deficit problems.

However, the real purpose for the breaks is to aid learning. People remember the first and the last things—educators call this the primacy and recency effect. More breaks mean more "firsts" and "lasts" to make an impression on one's brain.

Classroom content

New graduate content

When new graduates are asked about their biggest fears and concerns, they mention concerns about how to handle their many responsibilities (during school they only had to deal with one or two patients), how to handle emergencies (especially a "code"), and how to communicate with physicians / when to call the doctor.

The first step in teaching critical thinking may be to help them develop a plan of action to enable more effective responses when encountering these issues in practice. This will free up their energy to allow them to focus on the subtle patient-care assessments and important interventions.

Use some of these tips as a starting point for discussion.

Getting work done
- Provide a cheat sheet form for taking report or for the day's organization.

- Set "drop dead" times within your day (such as "all 9 a.m. medications to be in the patients' bodies by 9:30 a.m.") as guideposts for your progress in the day's time management.

- Work ahead. Always assume the unexpected will happen—it does.

- Keep current with your charting. It is harder to recall everything at the end of the day.

- Constantly reprioritize. Don't ask yourself, "What are all the things I should do?" but "What is most important for me to do?"

Emergencies/code
- Get help. For a code, if nothing else, go out in the hall and say, "I need help right now in room X!" in an urgent tone, with a loud, calm voice.

- Memorize the Institute for Healthcare Improvement (IHI) or other guidelines for activating a Rapid Response Team (see reference in resources section of Chapter 9). The IHI and other organizations have established recognized criteria for dealing with patients who could be critical and deteriorating. If anyone criticizes being contacted, cite the higher authority. "Well, the IHI indicates a Rapid Response Team should be activated for a sustained blood pressure below 90 systolic, so I felt it was advisable to follow the national criteria and get additional assistance."

Contacting the physician
- Take the initiative and introduce yourself to the physicians who admit frequently to your unit.

- Rehearse introductory statements/scripts for common needs. "Your patient (name) in room X is reporting Y and requesting Z. Do you want to order anything at this time?"

General advice
- Be slow to join a clique
- Make friends with the unit secretary

- Make your rounds during the night whether others do or not

- Make your own list of procedures or skills you have never experienced and let everyone on the unit (especially during orientation) know your desire to watch/participate in these tasks.

Teach in the context of clinical application

When planning a critical-thinking class for new graduates, experienced nurses, or both, remember that your session will be enhanced when the classroom time is spent applying knowledge to the clinical setting. Do not simply give a theory lecture. Instead, use images from books or sample labs. For example, you could hold up a picture of purpura and ask, "What do you think when you walk in and your patient looks like this?" Or present lab results (see below) and ask which value nurses should take care of first.

Value	Result	Normals
Glucose	193 mg/dL	70–110 mg/dL
BUN	8 mg/dL	10–20 mg/dL
Cr	0.7 mg/dL	0.7–1.2 mg/dL
Sodium	131 mEq/dL	136–145 mEq/dL
Potassium	3.2 mEq/dL	3.5–5.0 mEq/dL
SGOT/ALT	1932 IU/L	13–40 IU/L
SGPT/AST	2360 IU/L	7–60 IU/L
Bilirubin total	2.9 mg/dL	0.2–1.2 mg/dL

Experienced nurses are likely to pick potassium, but new graduate nurses rarely do so. Nurses learn the importance of potassium levels, in part, from work experience. This exercise will shorten the learning curve. You can also ask additional questions, such as

- What disease does the patient have?

- How does the patient look?

- Why isn't the sodium level the most important since it is "lower" than the potassium deficiency?

Prioritization

Nurses not only need to know what to do, but the importance and order in which things should be done. Nurses of all experience levels may need help with prioritization for multiple needs within one patient, between multiple patients, and between patient and administrative needs.

 ## Case study: Prioritization doesn't always come naturally

At one associate-degree nursing program, the faculty had assumed students would naturally pick up the concepts of prioritization. The faculty was appalled when the students scored below the national average in this category on a standardized test.

To remedy the problem, the nursing program added classroom time to talk about principles of prioritization, which was followed by a year-long integration of such principles into future content. By giving the problem a specific focus and emphasis, the school's students now score above national average in prioritization.

The handout developed for the second-year students can be found at the end of this chapter (Figure 3.1). This tool can either be used during critical-thinking classes, or given to attendees as a take-home reminder.

Strategies to teach prioritization

One way to teach prioritization principles is to use sample test questions dealing with prioritization, followed by a discussion of the rationale. For example:

Question: It is most important for the nurse to care for which patient complaint first?

    a.   Patient with type II diabetes mellitus with an a.m. blood sugar of 190mg.

    b.   Patient with a K+ of 3.2mEq who is receiving a K+ rider IVPB and states his arm is sore.

    c.   Patient with asthma treated with high-dose steroids states he is catching the "flu"; temperature is 100.4°F (38°C).

    d.   Patient with pneumonia being treated with IV antibiotics for one day. Today's WBC is 14,000mm^3.

Answer: The intended answer is C because immunocompromised patients present with suppressed symptoms. Follow-up discussion could include the difference if A was hypoglycemic, normal side effects of potassium infusions, and the fact that D is already being treated. However, discussion should also include the need to look at trends. If this was the patient's third day on antibiotics and the WBC is the same or increasing, we need to initiate action toward consideration of changing antibiotics.

First rule out the worst-case scenario

Everyone is influenced by what he or she sees most often or most recently. When dealing with a patient presentation, nurses must learn how to rule out the most lethal possible cause first.

One way is to indicate a patient condition seen frequently on the unit or department where the nurses in the particular class work, such as a one-day postoperative hip replacement. Ask the attendees what is essential for the nurse to do today. Common responses will likely include manage the pain, check the operative dressing, assess bowel and breath sounds, check the hemoglobin, watch the IV site and urine output, and verify PT is initiated.

Next ask what are the worst-case scenarios (i.e., most lethal complication) that could happen with this patient. How would you know if the patient was having those conditions? Discuss shock (possible loss of two liters in the hip), severe anemia (requiring transfusion), aspiration pneumonia, bowel ileus, sepsis, loss of circulation to the leg, dislocation of the prostethesis, or a secondary condition (myocardial infarction). Often, just the technique of bringing known material into the nurses' conscious awareness helps the process become second nature.

Use test questions and illustrative stories

Another strategy is to use test questions related to a patient presentation, and find out whether nurses assess for the worst-case scenario.

Question: A 96-year-old patient admitted with pneumonia is found crawling out of the bed. What should nurses do first?

    a.   Assess the patient's pain level.

    b.   Obtain a pulse oximeter reading.

    c.   Call for an order for a sedative.

    d.   Apply a Posey jacket.

Answer: Before you give the correct answer, B, talk about elderly patients' inability to compensate and how the brain is the most sensitive indicator for most things (low glucose, cerebral edema, etc.) Discuss whether they would feel tempted to answer differently if the person was 50 years old. Is the stereotype about all elderly people being a little confused influencing them?

Continue the lesson with a further illustration: A student nurse was told by another nurse to restrain the elderly person, which he did, but then the student nurse checked the pulse oximeter on his own. The patient was 86%.

Another true example of the danger of assuming all elderly people are confused: An elderly patient's daughter stated her mother was more confused than usual. Though the patient's pulse oximeter was 90%, no action was taken till the patient had a small stroke the next day. Diagnostics tests then revealed a small pulmonary embolism and a new stroke caused by a second clot.

Students remember stories—use them to get your point across.

New graduate nurses and more-experienced nurses who lack critical thinking skills tend to focus on the immediate task and orders rather than what should be done in the bigger picture. They fear acts of commission, such as giving the wrong medication. In doing so, they often commit acts of omission—not doing what they should do.

To train nurses how to focus on the bigger picture, start with common situations and discuss as a group what nurses should do:

- The patient has decreased pulses in his or her leg after a knee replacement. The nurse calls the resident, who reassures the nurse that the situation is fine. What should the nurse do when obtaining the same assessment two hours later?

- The patient has neuro checks ordered every two hours. The checks have been fine for the previous eight hours. It is now 2:00 a.m. and the patient is sleeping. What should the nurse do?

Often, inexperienced nurses focus on "assessing" because they are told to assess before acting. However, emphasize the need to act when they sense through assessment that something serious is wrong. Examples of actual legal cases help illustrate this point:

- A nurse charted that the patient's pulse remained 120 all night every hour on the hour, but did nothing (until the patient coded from internal hemorrhage).

- A nurse did not wake up the patient for a neuro assessment since the ABCs were stable, and the patient had some paralysis the following morning from cauda equina.

- A patient's pulse oximeter remained 80% after the physician checked the patient at 1:00 a.m. The patient coded at 6:00 a.m. with respiratory acidosis.

State how important it is to at least tell somebody. Emphasize that it is all right if nurses do not know the etiology or what treatment should be given. Discuss options if one person doesn't respond (such as the charge nurse, a colleague, the nursing supervisor, another resident, the attending physician, etc.).

Role-play what nurses should say in such situations, and remember that a little humility can go a long way. As Sylvia Rayfield (2002) suggests, start with "Help me to understand . . . "

Classroom processes

Repetition is the mother of all learning

Regardless of the style, new material needs reinforcement, and this is especially important for new graduates, as the anxiety of being new adds to the need to hear things more than once. When you teach, say something again, in a slightly different way. Use personal anecdotes, legal cases, or even published literature to illustrate the principle, emotions, and consequences of the lesson. The repetition and variety of methods are penetrating.

Use unfolding case scenarios

This technique is another way to incorporate the process of clinical critical thinking in a classroom setting. It provides the information in staggered amounts, punctuated by questions. The following are examples you can use.

The patient is a two-day postoperative hemi-colonectomy and asks for something for pain. Ask the attendees, "What is essential for the nurse to ask?" You have already decided ahead of time that the patient will have a more atypical problem, such as cholelithiasis from the anesthesia and dehydration or bladder distention after the catheter is removed, so respond appropriately to the questions the nurses ask. Don't let the "patient" tell the learners "giveaway" symptoms. Keep going until the learners specify where the pain is and palpate a positive Murphy's sign or distended bladder.

A 40-year-old presents with chest discomfort. The "patient" should also either be a cocaine user, an atypical cardiac presentation, or a smoker on birth control with a small pulmonary embolism. Did the attendees ask about drug use, prematurely rule out cardiac etiology due to the sex and age, and/or remember to check a pulse oximeter? Remind them to use incidence and "classic" presentations to help rule in considerations, but not to absolutely rule out.

Instructional approach and style

Cooperative learning

A growing trend in education is to have students teach students because "he who teaches, learns the most." One way to do this is the "think, pair, and share" exercise. Learners are given the general question and provided one minute to think about it and write down their thoughts. The task could be something like, "What are the three most important things to assess for in the first day on an abdominal postoperative patient?" or "What is something that makes it easier to delegate to an aide?"

After the minute is up, the participants then pair up and share their answers. Require each person to verbalize their thoughts to their partner, rather than just agreeing with the first person's statements. After time to share, one person is chosen as the spokesperson for the duo. Use a random selector to decide who shares, such as the person with the earliest birthday in the year, so both pay attention during the sharing.

Have the spokespeople stand and randomly select a few to repeat information from the paired sharing. Another way to change the selection is to use a version of musical chairs, passing a blown-up balloon, or have everyone stand and sit down according to certain criteria.

The advantage of a "think, pair, and share" exercise is that everyone participates. It accommodates those learners who initially need more time to think or have trouble speaking before others. They have rehearsed what they will say and can choose to enhance their response with their partners' comments. You also facilitate interaction with the material because participants must conceive it, write it, speak it, hear it, and work with it.

Multi-sensory learning

Most learning occurs through visual means, then hearing, with some touch. We all have our preferred style, but everyone will learn best when the logical left side and artistic right side of the brain are engaged.

Make sure your class varies the methods used to ensure multi-sensory learning. It's been shown that retention goes up to 50% when you hear and see something.

Effective use of discussion questions for class interaction

Throughout all discussions, pose good questions to stimulate thinking. Questions include, How does that work? What does that mean? What is the worst-case scenario here? What else do you need to know to make a decision? What makes this presentation different from the ordinary presentation? What do you want to do next? Why?

Another tip is to use silence. It can be tempting to jump in with the answer to fill the quiet (often awkward) moment that follows after a question. Train yourself to wait 10 seconds to allow time for the learners to respond. Tell the audience why you are waiting. Literally count off your fingers because 10 seconds can seem like an eternity.

It can be particularly effective to wait and not respond even when the right answer is given. This prevents learners from becoming good at reading the instructor rather than thinking about the issue. Alternatives include confirming the answer, but asking the person to defend it or to play the devil's advocate with the correct answer.

In the teaching scenarios, break the information down to what is essential, and also compare similarities or differences with a known concept. "How is this different from . . . ?"

Exude passion, as well as purpose

William Arthur Ward said, "The mediocre teacher tells. The good teacher explains. The superior teacher demonstrates. The great teacher inspires." The key behind great, effective teaching is not knowledge or methodology. It is holding a genuine passion for the material and for teaching.

When teaching, pull in emotion: We often forget what we think, but almost always remember how something made us feel. The teacher's excitement and belief about the material and its importance is infectious. The learner will either catch it or (at least) respect it.

References

Raines, C. 2002. "Managing Generation X Employees" in P. G. Zimmermann, *Nursing Management Secrets*. Philadelphia: Hanley & Belfus.

Rayfield, S., and L. Manning. 2002. *Nursing Made Insanely Easy!*, 3rd ed. Gulf Shore, AL: ICAN.

Salter, C. 2001. "16 ways to be a smarter teacher." *The Fast Company* 53: 114–126.

Shore, D. A., and P. G. Zimmerman. 1997. "Marketing your continuing education program." *Journal of Emergency Nursing* 23 (4): 363–366.

Zimmermann, P. G. and R. D. Herr. 2006. *Triage Nursing Secrets*. St. Louis: Mosby/Elsevier.

Zimmermann, P. G. 2006. "Writing effective test questions to measure triage competency: Tips for making a good triage test." *Journal of Emergency Nursing* 32 (1): 106–109.

Zimmermann, P. G. 2006. "Education and Training for Triage Nurses." In P. G. Zimmermann and R. D. Herr, *Triage Nursing Secrets*. St. Louis: Elsevier.

Zimmermann, P. G. 2003. "Orienting ED nurses to triage: Using scenario-based test-style questions to promote critical thinking." *Journal of Emergency Nursing* 29 (3): 256–258.

Zimmermann, P. G. 2003. "Some practical tips for more effective teaching." *Journal of Emergency Nursing* 29 (3): 283–286.

Zimmermann, P. G. 2002. "Guiding principles at triage: Advice for new triage nurses." *Journal of Emergency Nursing* 28 (1): 24–33.

Zimmermann, P. G. 2002. "The difference between teaching nursing students and registered nurses." *Journal of Emergency Nursing* 28 (6): 574—578.

Sources for example cases

- Legal case of the month from the Nurses Service Organization, available at *www.nso.com/case*

- Triage Column/Case Review/Clinical Educator in the *Journal of Emergency Nursing*

- Glendon, K., and D. Ulrich. 2001. *Unfolding Cases: Experiencing the Realities of Clinical Nursing Practice.* Upper Saddle River, NJ: Prentice Hall.

Figure 3.1	*Teaching critical thinking—Critical thinking course content and prioritization handout*

PRIORITIZATION HANDOUT

Determining the need

Two components: history and physical assessment

History

Be disciplined to be consistent and thorough. Consider using a mnemonic.

POSHPATE: History of the chief complaint (Rutenberg, C. 2000. "Telephone Triage." *American Journal of Nursing* 100(3):77-78, 80-81.)

P	Problem
O	Onset
S	Associated Symptoms
H	Previous History
P	Precipitating factors
A	Alleviating/Aggravating factors
T	Timing
E	Etiology

- Document key findings that allowed you to rule out the worst-case scenario or that made you think there was a problem.

- Compare to the patient's normal, especially for a chronic or elderly condition. ("You look like you are having a little trouble breathing. Is that how you are feeling?")

- Your concern should be heightened if the patient is concerned enough to complain about an "ordinary" condition (e.g., headache).

Figure

3.1

Teaching critical thinking—Critical thinking course content and prioritization handout (cont.)

Assess before acting

Question: One-day postoperative patient complains of pain. Nurses should first

a. administer the ordered prn analgesic

c. obtain a description of the pain

b. assess for the presence of bowel sounds

d. check the vital signs

Answer: C. Do not assume the pain is postoperative. Postoperative patients can have MIs or cholecystitis.

Prioritization with individual patients

Maslow

Self-actualization needs

Esteem needs

Safety needs

Physiologic needs

ABCD: A before B before C before D

A Airway	If the patient is talking, the airway is intact
B Breathing	Normal respirations are quiet and effortless
C Circulation	Pink, warm, orientation r/t perfusion
D Disability	Pain
	Neurological assessment
	Mental status changes

Quick Tip: 30-2-CAN DO means patient is adequately oxygenated and perfused to allow you to proceed. (Respirations are less than 30, oriented to person and place, obeys commands.)

Among ABCD, level of severity is considered.

 Critical Thinking in the Emergency Department

Figure 3.1   *Teaching critical thinking—Critical thinking course content and prioritization handout (cont.)*

Question: All of these patients complain of being short of breath. Which patient should nurses provide care to first?

    a. Patient with bronchitis who can speak phrases

    b. Patient with emphysema with a PO2 of 92% on 2L/min

    c. Patient three days post-operative with a cough productive of green phlegm

    d. Patient with asthma on whom the nurse cannot auscultate breath sounds

Answer: D

AIRWAY

Risk for airway problems

- Decreased level of consciousness
- Sedated
- Vomiting
- Allergic reactions (unpredictable progression)

Signs of airway distress

- Hoarseness (after smoke inhalation, unrelated to a cold)
- Singed nasal hairs
- Snoring respirations (tongue falling back in an unconscious patient)
- Presence of vomitus, bleeding, secretions
- Edema of the lips/mouth tissues
- Preferred position (tripod)
- Drooling in an adult (throat is too swollen to swallow spit, epiglottis)
- Dysphagia
- Abnormal signs, such as strider, burgling, "death rattle" from secretions

Assess

- Look, listen, feel
- Level of consciousness r/t oxygenation

Teaching critical thinking—Critical thinking course content and prioritization handout (cont.)

Interventions

- Reposition

- Suction

BREATHING

Assess

- Respiration rate AND depth

- Symmetrical chest rise and fall

- Presence and quality of bilateral breath sounds

- Pulse oximeter

Signs of respiratory problems

- Increased work of breathing (nasal flaring, retractions, expiratory grunting, accessory muscle use, head bobbing)

- Paradoxical respirations

- Jugular vein distention

- Tracheal position

- Abnormal breath sounds (silent chest is the most ominous because air is not moving)

- Color, especially circumoral (cyanosis is a late sign)

- Lack of integrity in chest wall

- Speaks in words, phrases, incomplete sentences

| Figure 3.1 | Teaching critical thinking—Critical thinking course content and prioritization handout (cont.) |

Related routine aspects to assess

• Is incentive spirometer within the patient's reach? Can/does the patient use it properly and frequently enough?

• Is oxygen on properly, correct amount?

• Peak flow

• Patient's self-rating on the work of the breathing (Borg scale)

Interventions
• Position
• Oxygen
• Ventilation

CIRCULATION

Assess
• Skin color, temperature
• Perfusion through blanching, capillary refill
• Pulse: rate, rhythm characteristics

General rule of thumb: Adults with a radial pulse have $\geq$ 80 systolic (brachial $\geq$ 70; jugular $\geq$ 60); low perfusion; respiratory and heart rate increase first, before blood pressure

Blood pressure: Adults must lose about 1500cc; children about 25% of volume before hypotension onsets

Figure

3.1

Teaching critical thinking—Critical thinking course content and prioritization handout (cont.)

Signs of circulation difficulties

- Early signs and symptoms: loss of consciousness (LOC)

- Children: loss of peripheral, then central pulses, extremity mottling

- Uncontrolled bleeding: spurting = arterial

- Distended jugular veins

- Distant heart tones

- Pitting dependent edema: pedal, sacral in a bedridden patient

- Most frequent sign of deep-vein thrombosis: unilateral extremity swelling

- Neurovascular (5 Ps)

  - Paresthesia is the early sign; nerves are more sensitive than pulse

Interventions

- IV

  - Is the site intact?

  - Is the dressing intact?

  - Is the infusion "working" at the proper rate?

- Drainage

  - Dressing dry and intact?

- Circulation devices (foot pumps, SCDs, TED hose properly applied)

DISABILITY

Assess

- Alteration of orientation x 3 (scales)

- Alertness

- Neuro checks (Glasgow Coma Scale, PERRLA, movement/strength in all extremities)

- Pain

  - Objective score.

  - PQRST.

  - Effect on normal ADL.

Figure

3.1

Teaching critical thinking—Critical thinking course content and prioritization handout (cont.)

- More concern if the pain wakes the patient up, reaches maximum intensity in the first minute, patient can recall the exact moment it started suddenly, or is similar to the pain the patient had for a serious etiology (e.g., "This feels like the last time I had a heart attack.").

- If patient states it is the "worst pain in my life" but appears comfortable or has a minor complaint (e.g., sore throat), ask about the person's previous worst pain experience. Any experience is the worst the first time you have it. If compared to significant event, such as childbirth, kidney stone, or broken bone, then accept it.

Assessment guidelines

Consider and rule out the worst-case scenario patients could have with this complaint.

What area or problem is most likely to result with this patient's condition?

Facial surgery	Airway/breathing
Broken arm	Compartment syndrome, loss of circulation
Diabetes	Hypoglycemia, DKA, HHNK
Abdominal surgery	Dehiscence, evisceration; shock; infection; bowel obstruction

Question: Which assessment is most important for a patient with a chest tube?

a. Respiratory rate

b. Pulse rate

c. Pain level

d. Temperature

Answer: A

Figure

3.1

Teaching critical thinking—Critical thinking course content and prioritization handout (cont.)

Question: An elderly patient is four days postoperative from abdominal surgery. Today the patient has a temperature of 103.1°F (39.5°C), 104/60, 110/20. This morning's WBC results are 20,000. It is most important for nurses to

a. administer a prn antipyretic

c. assess for bowel sounds

b. monitor the vital signs every hour

d. call the physician for antibiotics

Answer: D

Go for the most common problem first. "When you hear hoof beats, think horses, not zebras."

Question: The patient presents with a forearm deformity from falling 3 hours ago. He complains of severe pain.

What is the most likely explanation? Pain from a fracture

What must be ruled out? Compartment syndrome, loss of circulation

How will you assess this? 5 Ps; passive stretching, if relief obtained from analgesic

Patients before paperwork.

Stop any procedure causing harm.

Question: While the nurse is administering an IV antibiotic, the patient becomes flushed and complains of feeling hot. The nurses should first

a. complete an Adverse Drug Reaction form

b. call the doctor for an order for an antihistamine

c. stop the infusion

d. check the client's allergic history

Answer: C

 Critical Thinking in the Emergency Department

Figure
3.1

Teaching critical thinking—Critical thinking course content and prioritization handout (cont.)

Question: The charge nurse notices the new nursing assistant placing the patient's urine Foley bag on a hook at the height of the patient's chest. What is the best response for the nurse to make?

a. Move the bag and speak to the assistant now.

b. Speak to the nursing assistant at the end of the shift.

c. Discuss the need for additional inservicing with the nurse educator.

d. Write an incident report and inform the nurse manager.

Answer: A

Medications tend to be a priority, especially for anti-diabetic and antibiotic medications because of the lack of effectiveness if not given in a timely manner.

Question: The patient is admitted from the emergency department with a diagnosis of bacterial meningitis. Which of the following orders is most important for the nurse to do first?

a. Obtain a set of vital signs.

b. Administer the IV antibiotic.

c. Perform a neuro assessment

d. Administer the prn antipyretic.

Answer: B

Consider the timing/type of medication

Two antibiotics are ordered for 1:00 p.m. One is every 24 hours, one is every 4 hours. The nurse should administer the one ordered every 4 hours first at 1:00 pm to allow for the best interval.

<table>
<tr><td>*Figure*
3.1</td><td>*Teaching critical thinking—Critical thinking
course content and prioritization handout (cont.)*</td></tr>
</table>

Question: A nurse had been involved with an emergency on the patient unit and is late in administering the team's 9:00 a.m. medications. Which of the 9:00 a.m. medications is most important for the nurse to administer first?

a. Ampicillin 1000mg IVPB every 6 hours

b. Vancomycin 1 gram IVPB every 36 hours

c. Lanoxin (Digoxin) 0.125mg daily

d. Aspirin 81mg daily

Answer: A

Question: A nurse was involved with another patient's cardiac arrest and is behind schedule with medications. It is now 8:00 a.m. Which medication is most important?

a. Colace

b. Ferrous sulfate

c. Erythromycin po

d. 70/30 insulin

Answer: D

Prioritization principles

Acute before chronic.

Question: Which of the following patients is most important for the nurse to follow up with first?

a. Reports unilateral blurry central vision for one year.

b. States has a veil starting to come across the vision in one eye.

c. Yellow discharge noted from right eye, relates had it for one day.

d. Complains of itching eyes during the spring.

Answer: B

Sudden onset is usually more serious than gradual onset. Actual over potential.

| Figure 3.1 | Teaching critical thinking—Critical thinking course content and prioritization handout (cont.) |

Trends

- **Any symptom associated with other definitive changes** (e.g., not feeling well, and a fever, and feeling short of breath)

- **Any minor symptoms that tend to recur repeatedly or intensify in severity** ("nagging" cough that won't go away, smoker)

- **Steady progressive decline**

Question: Which patient with these findings is most important for the nurse to check on first?

a. Respirations: 16, 18, 20

b. Radial pulse: 80, 86, 92

c. Blood pressure: 150/80, 130/78, 110/70

d. Pulse oximeter: 99%, 97%, 96%

Answer: C

Life before limb (systemic before local).

Question: Which patient should the nurse take care of first?

a. Patient with Billroth II procedure complaining of incisional discomfort rated "6."

b. Patient with deep-vein thrombosis complaining of shortness of breath.

c. Patient with low-back pain complaining that it radiates down the right leg.

d. Patient with chronic arterial insufficiency complaining of leg pain while walking.

Answer: B

Patient demographics

Presence of other risk factors increase this patient's priority

- Elderly (decreased immunity, decreased reserves to fight other stresses)
- Very young (decreased immunity)
- Altered immunity (leukemia, HIV+ or AIDS, taking steroids, splenectomy)
- Transplanted organs (risk of electrolyte imbalance, immunosuppressed)
- Multiple comorbidities (especially diabetes because less immunity)
- Pregnancy (risk to fetus)
- Reaction that has a potential to worsen (overdose, allergic response)

Avoid exposure of susceptible individuals.

Question: The unit will receive a new admission from the emergency department diagnosed with bacterial pneumonia. Which of the following patients would be the best choice for a roommate?

a. 19-year-old with diabetic ketoacidosis (DKA)

b. 80-year-old who had abdominal surgery

c. 15-year-old with a broken leg in traction.

d. 60-year-old stroke victim with right-sided paralysis

Answer: C

Remember a "known" patient can develop a new problem

Figure
3.1

Teaching critical thinking—Critical thinking course content and prioritization handout (cont.)

Avoid the "Oh my GOD!" distracter (red herring)

Question: A nurse decides to help out when coming upon a head-on collision car accident that just occurred. The nurse notes the victim has bright red blood spurting from the shoulder and a detached arm is lying at the patient's side. The right leg is turned 180 degrees, facing backwards. The nurse should first

    a. apply direct pressure to the source of the spurting blood.

    b. assess for a pedal pulse in the deformed leg.

    c. check for a carotid pulse

    d. verify that the airway is open.

Answer: D

Remember to avoid WHO rather than "what"

Just because someone is more demanding or "ranked" higher should not distract from a more urgent patient need. Express your limit. "I understand you need me. I have to take care of this urgent need first and then I can work with you."

Question: Which of the following should the nurse take care of first?

    a. The bathroom sink has a leak.

    b. An irate family member is in the hall, demanding to see the supervisor.

    c. A patient is lying on the floor, having fallen and hit her head.

    d. A physician is at the nurse's station and wants to discuss an order.

Answer: C

Remember, prioritization does not mean a person's need is not met. It is first things first so the right care is given to the right person at the right time for the right reason.

Source: Polly Gerber Zimmermann, RN, MS, MBA, CEN

Figure

3.2

Teaching critical thinking skills—
Sample course content, objectives, and agenda

SAMPLE COURSE CONTENT

Sample course objectives

1. Identify four mechanisms or thought processes that are examples of critical thinking.

2. List two validations for the need of accurate baseline assessments.

3. Describe the hospital policy on patient reassessments.

4. Relate an atypical geriatric patient scenario that involves the cardiopulmonary system.

5. Identify two medications commonly prescribed to the geriatric patient that may mask signs/symptoms of shock.

6. Relate two responsibilities of the nurse that require critical thinking skills.

7. Describe the use of pertinent negatives and positives in nursing documentation.

Sample course content

- Patient assessment
  - Reviewing collected data and making a decision
  - Using pertinent negatives and positives
  - Common errors
  - How vital are vital signs?

- Documentation
  - When to document

| *Figure* 3.2 | ***Teaching critical thinking skills—*** *** Sample course content, objectives, and agenda (cont.)*** |

- What not to document
- Where to document

• When to call the physician
   - Age-specific concerns

• Red flags of assessment
   - Case scenarios

• Incorporating policy and procedure

• Professional responsibilities
   - Scope of practice
   - Risk management

Sample scenarios for student workbook or discussion

Case 1

Temp 97.4° (rectal)   Pulse 118   Respirations 26   Blood Pressure 128/72

Which vital sign is not only out of the normal range, but of most concern to you?

What are you concerned about with this adult patient?

What should you assess on this patient to determine if there is a potential for demise?

Case 2

Temp 102.4° (oral)   Pulse 78   Respirations 14   Blood Pressure 78/52

In the adult patient, what is of concern to you with these vital signs?

What other information do you need to determine if there is a potential for demise?

Source: Shelley Cohen, RN, BS, CEN

Figure

3.3

Teaching critical thinking skills—
Classroom tips

TIPS FOR A SUCCESSFUL CLASS

1. Incorporate anatomy and physiology

- Hand out crayons or colored pencils

- Use applicable anatomy sheets from *www.enchantedlearning.com*

- Display (slide or poster) the anatomy section you want them to fill in

- Identify a specific area (for example, the brain) and have them color it a certain color)

- When completed, display a correct completed anatomy picture and have learners self-correct their drawings

2. Incorporate policy and procedures

- Identify policy/procedure appropriate to case scenarios you are using
- Ask if they know where to retrieve/access the policy/procedure
- Emphasize standards of practice

3. Case scenarios

- Use as many as you can fit into the time period
- If multiple specialty areas are in the class, vary the scenarios
- Relate critical-thinking strategies as you go through the cases

4. Documentation

- Use your standard nursing documentation forms or a printout of your electronic form

Figure 3.3	Teaching critical thinking skills— Classroom tips (cont.)

- Give them a case scenario and have them document the patient assessment
- Go around the room and have a few participants read their charts
- Display a correct documentation note for the patient case
- Discuss risk-management concerns related to documentation

5. Resources

- If you can access the Internet in your classroom setting, search for clinical scenarios that have photos (e.g., a rash, EKG and pose questions to the participants)

- Use tools such as crossword puzzles to help participants improve their prioritizing skills

6. Evaluation

Obtain feedback from participants to determine if they would like a follow-up to this critical thinking–skills course. Give them course content options and let them check off which they are interested in:

- More anatomy and physiology
- Laboratory results
- IV fluids
- Critical situation scenarios
- Interventions for an emergency

7. Self assessment tools

Incorporate a self-assessment tool that participants can complete and use to work with preceptors or managers (Figure 3.4). Consider having them complete the same form before and after the class to validate the need for the course and to show them how attending has improved their critical thinking skills.

Source: Shelley Cohen, RN, BS, CEN

<table>
<tr><td>

Figure

3.4

</td><td>

Teaching critical thinking skills—
Sample self-assessment tool

</td></tr>
</table>

CRITICAL THINKING SELF-ASSESSMENT

Use the following scale to respond to each statement:

4 = I feel very comfortable with this

3 = I feel somewhat comfortable with this

2 = I feel somewhat uncomfortable with this

1 = I feel very uncomfortable with this

1.	Calling the physician at 3 a.m. regarding a patient's status	4	3	2	1
2.	Identifying a patient at risk for an immediate demise	4	3	2	1
3.	Initiating emergency measures until help arrives	4	3	2	1
4.	Relating changes in vital signs to the individual patient scenario	4	3	2	1
5.	Knowing when to bring a patient-care concern to the attention of the charge nurse / team leader	4	3	2	1
6.	Identifying age-specific red flags that would alert me to reassess the patient	4	3	2	1
7.	Knowing what to document and what not to document	4	3	2	1
8.	Identifying patient situations that may be a risk for myself or the organization	4	3	2	1
9.	Verbally relaying to another professional my concerns regarding a patient's status	4	3	2	1

Source: Shelley Cohen, RN, BS, CEN

Figure

3.5

Teaching critical thinking skills—Handout

Sample pocket card. Print out, fold in half, laminate (if possible), and give to attendees of the critical thinking class.

Attributes of a critical thinker	**When to call the provider**
• Asks pertinent questions	• Perfusion problem
• Assesses statements and arguments	• Pain issue
• Is curious about things	• Standing-order concern
• Listens to others and is able to give feedback	• Atypical presentation complaints
• Looks for evidence or proof	• Risk-management potential
• Examines problems closely	• What's going in isn't coming out
• Can reject information that is not relevant or is incorrect	• Negative response to intervention
• Wants to find the solution	• Social concerns / family issues affecting patient care
• Thinks independently	
• Questions deeply	
• Has intellectual integrity	
• Is confident in rationale for actions	
• Analyzes arguments	
• Evaluates evidence and facts	
• Explores consequences before taking action	
• Recognizes a contradiction	
• Evaluates policy	

Reference: Ferrett, S. 1997. *Peak Performance: Success in College and Beyond.* New York: McGraw-Hill.

Source: Shelley Cohen, RN, BS, CEN

Orientation: Bringing critical thinking to the clinical environment

Moving from the classroom to the bedside

As educators and nurse leaders start to think about developing a process to move teaching critical thinking from the classroom to the work setting, consider these questions:

- Can nurses who learn critical thinking in the classroom setting apply it in the clinical environment?

- How do you evaluate their ability to apply this knowledge?

- Does your orientation process incorporate critical thinking and how you do a baseline assessment on the new staff you hire?

- Are experienced nursing staff given the education they need so they may learn to identify key opportunities to develop critical thinking in your new staff?

If you focus on critical thinking from the beginning of orientation through to the annual review process, nurses will understand the vital role it plays in delivering safe patient care. Incorporating critical thinking into ongoing orientation processes allows you to build a nursing culture that embraces the concept of critical thinking from the date of hire.

Beginning with orientation

When you mention orientation to a new nursing staff members they typically think of sitting in a classroom to learn specifics about your organization. They expect you to address medication policies, fire safety, and the Joint Commission on Accreditation of Healthcare Organizations (JCAHO), among other regulatory requirements. They also expect to take a medication test to validate that they can apply their skills in the clinical arena.

Since nurses know these items will be addressed as part of the orientation process, this is an ideal setting to introduce your expectations on critical thinking abilities, both for new graduate nurses and for those with more experience.

Self-assessment

Once orientees have undergone classroom education regarding critical thinking, they will naturally conduct their own internal review of the information to figure out how well they function with the concepts. It is to be expected that new graduate nurses will demonstrate the most hesitancy in this area.

Regardless of the years of experience of your new hires, conducting a self assessment is a valuable tool to measure their perception of their ability to perform at the critical-thinking level. Figure 4.1, on page 55, is an example of a tool that can be used to measure nurses' critical thinking skills for general nursing responsibilities. Figure 4.2, on page 57, is tailored for ED-specific skills during the ED part of orientation. Give either or both of these forms to new hires to complete at the start of orientation. The forms should be reviewed by the new hires and by their preceptors, and occasionally even their managers.

| Figure | Critical thinking self-assessment tool— |
| 4.1 | General nursing skills |

Employee name: _____

Date of hire: _____

Position hired for: _____

This self-assessment tool will help guide your preceptor and manager throughout your orientation process to ensure we provide you with the tools and resources you need for success.

How comfortable are you at doing the things listed below?

	I feel very comfortable with this	I feel somewhat comfortable with this	I feel somewhat uncomfortable with this	I feel very uncomfortable with this	Comments
Calling the doctor at 3:00 a.m. about a patient's status					
Identifying a patient at risk for immediate demise					
Initiating emergency measures until help arrives					
Identifying possible causes of vital sign changes related to the patient's condition					

Figure
4.1

Critical thinking self-assessment tool— General nursing skills (cont.)

	I feel very comfortable with this	I feel somewhat comfortable with this	I feel somewhat uncomfortable with this	I feel very uncomfortable with this	Comments
Knowing when to bring a patient-care concern to the attention of the charge nurse					
Identifying age-specific alerts that indicate the patient needs reevaluation					
Knowing what to document and what not to document					
Identifying patient scenarios that may be a risk-management concern					
Verbally relaying concerns to another professional					

Source: Shelley Cohen, RN, BS, CEN

| Figure | Critical thinking self-assessment tool— |
| 4.2 | Emergency nursing skills |

Employee name: _____

Date of hire: _____

Position hired for: _____

This self-assessment tool will help guide your preceptor and manager throughout your orientation process to ensure we provide you with the tools and resources you need for success.

How comfortable are you at doing the things listed below?

	I feel very comfortable with this	I feel somewhat comfortable with this	I feel somewhat uncomfortable with this	I feel very uncomfortable with this	Comments
Identifying red flags that a patient is not perfusing well					
Defining my role when a patient has a critical lab value					
Making a decision at triage that reflects the seriousness of the presentation					
Anticipating needs of patients presenting with commonly seen emergencies					

Figure 4.2	Critical thinking self-assessment tool— Emergency nursing skills (cont.)				
	I feel very comfortable with this	I feel somewhat comfortable with this	I feel somewhat uncomfortable with this	I feel very uncomfortable with this	Comments
Identifying nonverbal clues that my patient may be a victim of violence					
Recognizing signals that a patient or visitor has the potential for violent behavior					
Redirecting the ED physician to the patient in greatest need of intervention					

Source: Shelley Cohen, RN, BS, CEN

When developing your own self-assessment tool, or adapting the ones included, make sure to include items that reflect

- generic nursing skill
- specialty-area questions
- questions for both the novice and experienced nurse

New hires should be asked to complete the same self-assessment tools when they conclude their orientation period, or after about three months. You can then compare the responses to the initial assessment, which also could be reviewed by the preceptor and/or manager. Keep in mind that the responses may show no difference when the experience or knowledge level of nurses is at its peak performance level. Others should show marked improvements during this period, particularly new graduate nurses.

Having new employees conduct a self-assessment at the beginning of orientation and again after they have been at your facility for a few months helps by

- clarifying and defining their critical thinking abilities and identifying areas that require more attention during orientation

- providing a documentation process that validates areas of strength and weakness

- becoming a resource tool from which you and the nurse may develop goals

- providing a record of the dates that orientees demonstrated these proficiencies

The role of preceptors

As new hires transition through the orientation process, their assigned preceptors will be key to the application of critical thinking in the clinical practice area. Regardless of experience level, new hires will look to their preceptors as role models for critical thinking skills.

Before preceptors can teach critical thinking to orientees, they must first be practicing the skills themselves. Therefore, make sure you pick clinically competent critical thinkers who will be suitable role models for the type of nursing care you want practiced. It is also important that the organization invest time and education in training preceptors so they can meet your expectations.

Preceptors should be provided with guidelines and goals to follow as they orient new employees. This will help them to

- validate successful goals in the new hire

- clearly identify areas that require remediation

- present organized documentation to show that the new hire is able to meet the requirements of the job for which they were hired

New hires who quickly display critical thinking skills will bring a great sense of relief to their preceptors. All new hires should display skills as they progress through their development, but those who show evidence earlier than others take quite a load off the mind of the preceptor.

How can preceptors teach critical thinking?

Preceptors can help orientees develop and stimulate the use of critical thinking skills by following some of these suggestions.

Minimizing the emphasis on ability to perform skills and tasks: New hires are eager to complete the required "check-offs" for competencies related to performing clinical tasks. Preceptors should encourage them to focus on other aspects of their orientation as well, for example, finding the facility's policy on dealing with patients who want to leave AMA.

Maximizing emphasis on the ability to recognize when the skill or task is needed: As new hires request to be "checked off" on various skills or tasks, preceptors should ask questions to demonstrate whether new hires have the ability to critically think through why the patient needs this particular task or skill performed.

Encourage a realistic time frame and expectations: Display time-related goals for the new hire so the peer group will not have unrealistic expectations of when the new hire will be comfortable with something. Post a spreadsheet that lists the names of the orientees and goals for the next 30 days. Affix dates to the items so preceptors may check them off when successfully completed. This serves to keep all staff up to date on what orientees are competent to do, and ensures they do not delegate a task for which an orientee is not yet prepared. It also keeps a check on any unrealistic expectations staff nurses may have for new hires. Staff nurses can look at the list and know that orientees cannot admit a patient on their own because that skill will not be taught until the next time sheet.

Do not assume the new hire understands the what, why, how, or when of delivering nursing care: If the orientee is a seasoned nurse, the preceptor should not make assumptions that length of experience is directly related to knowledge and ability to use critical thinking skills. Instead, all new hires should be required to demonstrate the same knowledge. The preceptor can use prompting questions to begin the what, why, how, and when questioning to allow the new hire to demonstrate appropriate reasoning.

Figure 4.3 serves as a helpful guide for both the preceptor and the orientee to validate this process of finding out the what, why, how, and when.

Figure 4.3	Preceptor tool—Relating skills to critical thinking for new graduate nurses

RELATING SKILLS TO CRITICAL THINKING

	Why does my patient need this?	How will I know if it is working?	What else should I consider/observe?	How long will my patient need it for?
Intravenous access				
Foley catheter				
Colostomy bag				
Dressing change				
Wound healing				
Splint application				
Bowel assessment				

Source: Shelley Cohen, RN, BS, CEN

Teachable moments

Once new hires are in the clinical setting, there are numerous opportunities for the preceptor to teach and demonstrate the application of critical thinking with actual patients. This is also the time when new hires to reveal their ability to apply the knowledge they started learning in the orientation classroom.

Examples of "teachable moments" include

- preparation of assignment/organization during their shift

- information shared during shift report

- early identification of patients in need of specific interventions that can involve new hires

- prompting the what/why/how/when questions for specific patient scenarios

Figure 4.4 is a tool to encourage the critical thinking of the orientee, and can be filled in to provide further examples of situations that present teachable moments. Adapt the problem list in this figure to include items directly related to your clinical practice area.

| Figure 4.4 | Preceptor tool—Relating patient observations to critical thinking |

DEALING WITH PROBLEMS AND SITUATIONS

Problem or situation	What does the patient need?	Why does the patient need this?	How do I do this?	When should I do this?	What should I document? Where do I document?
Patient fluid intake is poor					
Patient is complaining of abdominal pain					
Parent shows no remorse in delaying care of ill child					
Provider orders medication dose that is out of normal range					
Geriatric patient has an acute mental status change					
Lab calls a critical lab value to your attention					

Source: Shelley Cohen, RN, BS, CEN

Sometimes nursing staff other than the preceptor may be working with the orientee. During these times, it is essential that the preceptor educate all staff on the importance of their role in assisting with the transition process of the newly hired nurse.

The preceptor can promote and encourage positive behaviors among staff that will help to promote and motivate the critical thinking process. Figure 4.5 is a tool preceptors can share with other staff to encourage their understanding and support for developing new employees' critical thinking. It has essential reminders that include

- faster is not always clinically better

- checking things off for a new hire indicates you observed them perform it

- proactively involve new hires in challenging patient scenarios—but be there to support them

- ask prompting questions that validate they can apply knowledge

- knowing where your department resources are is as important as learning tasks and skills

| Figure 4.5 | *Preceptor tool—Promote and support critical thinking* |

EVERYONE CAN PROMOTE AND SUPPORT CRITICAL THINKING

To encourage newly hired nurses in their orientation process, we all need to provide a supportive and nurturing clinical environment. We want team members who can answer the what/why/how/when of nursing process.

Here's how you can help to create this environment.

1. **Faster is not necessarily better, as long as it's done correctly**

   Does it really matter—in many situations—if it takes new hires a few minutes longer to get in the IV? Yes, you could have done it faster—but how fast did you do it when you were a new nurse?

2. **Make no assumptions about skills**

   If you are asked to check off a new hire on a skill, be sure you actually observe the performance of this skill and then ask:

   - Why does/did this patient need a _____?
   - How did you know the correct way to perform this?
   - Where did you find the information?
   - How will you tell if the procedure is helpful for the patient?
   - What and where will you document what you have done?

3. **When you identify a challenging patient scenario or a procedure not commonly performed, invite the new hire to participate**

   This will help increase the experience of the new hire, as well as help the team identify the new hire's willingness to learn.

 Critical Thinking in the Emergency Department

Figure *4.5*	***Preceptor tool—Promote and*** ***support critical thinking (cont.)***

4. **At shift change report ask prompting questions in a non-defensive manner**

    - What do you think is going on with this patient?
    - Are you comfortable with what the provider told you after you spoke with him or her?

5. **Observe new hires' ability to prioritize and organize their assignments**

    - Is there a particular reason you have not done the pre-op teaching yet on Mrs. Jones?

    - You look concerned. Is everything ok? Let's go over your assignment and talk about priorities for the shift. I'd like to hear what you think are the most important issues in these patients and why.

6. **When questions arise, do they know where to look for the answers or are they simply expecting coworkers to answer them?**

    - I am not sure about these medicines being compatible. How could you find out?

    - When you are not sure whether a permit is needed for a procedure, where could you find that information?

Source: Shelley Cohen, RN, BS, CEN

Evaluating skills

As new nurses work their way through the orientation process, evaluating their ability to apply critical thinking in their clinical setting needs to be accomplished. Sometimes knowing what to do is as important as knowing what not to do. The preceptor needs evidence of new hires' abilities to assess the needs of each patient.

The following should be assessed:

- Evaluate a patient's health status: Are their patient assessment skills targeted to the patient's presentation?

- Identify potential scenarios based on the patient's health status: Are they aware of potential problems or complications this patient may be at risk for?

- Evaluate a patient's response to interventions: Are they performing an appropriate reassessment? Can they identify if the patient is the same, worse, or better?

- Evaluate the need for higher skill level: If patient is not responding to intervention, do they know what to do next?

- Take action when indicated: Can they initiate actions needed by patients, such as standing orders? Are they able to prioritize these actions?

Handling judgment or action errors during orientation

In any moment of decision the best thing to do is the right thing, the next best thing is the wrong thing, and the worst thing you can do is nothing.

—Theodore Roosevelt

It is more encouraging to see an orientee taking action in the clinical setting than those who elect to do nothing about a patient situation. The fact that they are willing to do something shows they are making progress. And the reality is that an error of judgment may be made by an experienced nurse as well as a new graduate.

It's important to understand that placing an experienced nurse in a new and unfamiliar clinical specialty area creates an opportunity for judgment or action errors, just as new graduates may make errors due to their unfamiliarity with nursing. Experienced nurses who have moved to a new clinical specialty will be exposed to unfamiliar medications, procedures, and possible age-specific considerations. For example, an experienced neonatal ICU nurse who transitions to the emergency department is going into a world that includes both adult and pediatric patients. The nurse's medication dosing was very different in the neonatal ICU setting than it will be for adult patients in the ED. In addition, he or she will experience different situations and interactions with patients. For the most part, he or she will not develop relationships with ED patients for more than a few hours and may never meet patients' families for any additional medical information.

Accept that errors will occur and lay the groundwork for making sure errors are handled in the correct manner. Preceptors and the entire peer group play a large role in the recovery process when errors occur, and should help ensure that incidents become an opportunity to develop critical thinking skills that will reduce such incidents in the future.

In addition, the response of the preceptor and peers to these scenarios will determine whether new hires feel supported during what is a challenging time for them. Nurses are often quick to "quarterback" incidents with comments about how "We would never have done that" or "I would never have done that first." Remember that orientation is a time of learning, setting goals, and identifying areas of strength and weakness. Newly hired nurses should not be left with a feeling of "being chewed up and spit out" by their peer group.

All incidents can be used as learning experiences. When errors occur, they may reveal some positive attributes about the new hire:

- The nurse was willing to be held accountable and identified the error to you

- The nurse was grateful and appreciative that you pointed out the error

- The nurse requested resources for self-learning to better understand the red flags that he or she missed with the patient

- The nurse asked questions to better understand how the patient got to this point

- The nurse sought guidance in completing a reporting form if one was needed

Preceptors or mentors of new employees must identify the decisions that were or were not made by the nurse that reflect a lack of critical thinking. Once these are recognized, then the preceptor can become the teacher to guide the nurse as he or she learns so that a similar situation is not replayed in the future.

Remediation

Working with new hires on remediation after an event is a delicate job. How you handle the situation will greatly affect how much they learn, how they feel and whether they can accept what happened, and whether they develop their critical thinking skills so as to understand the situation.

These teaching qualities will help you have a successful interaction:

Patience: What is obvious critical thinking to you may not be for others. You may need to provide repetition in the learning process and allow time for the nurse to digest the information before requiring him or her to demonstrate understanding.

Support: Being supportive after an error in judgment does not mean you minimize the importance of what occurred. It simply reflects that you support the nurse. Some words to use to send a supportive and reassuring message include

- I understand you are upset about what happened with Mr. Smith

- I realize this material is all new to you—let's go over it again

- Take a step back and look at all the things you have accomplished

- Good for you for recognizing and notifying me of the error—it takes courage and strong ethics to do so

Clarification: Define in writing for the new hire what you expect of him or her in light of what has occurred. If you discussed timelines, include those in the written expectations. For the new hire who simply does not have the capacity to apply critical thinking, it is essential that your documentation reflect what happened, what steps were taken, and what improvements were expected to occur so as to validate any future employment decisions. Examples of written expectations include

- all medication doses requiring calculations will be reviewed with the preceptor prior to administering to the patient.

- in the next two weeks, the orientee will demonstrate appropriate priorities for the patient presenting with a complaint of chest pain. Standing orders will be initiated per department policy.

- there will be no further incidents of patients signing out AMA without nursing documentation that "tells the story" of these events. The orientee will develop a list of other risk-management scenarios related to the department and present these at our next scheduled orientation meeting.

Realism: Keep in mind the reality of the situation. It is not about what you learned in nursing school or when you went through orientation years ago. It is about the present situation and the circumstances and experiences of the new nurse.

- Remember that not all new grads are clinically prepared at the same level

- Review critical thinking goals and timelines to ensure they are appropriate

- Recognize those nurses who may never be able to meet these goals successfully, and deal with the situation appropriately

Orientation sets critical-thinking expectations

The orientation process and critical thinking should go hand in hand. Orientation allows new hires to see how the critical thinking skills they learned in the classroom can be integrated into practice. It is the foundation upon which they can build on their development from novice to expert.

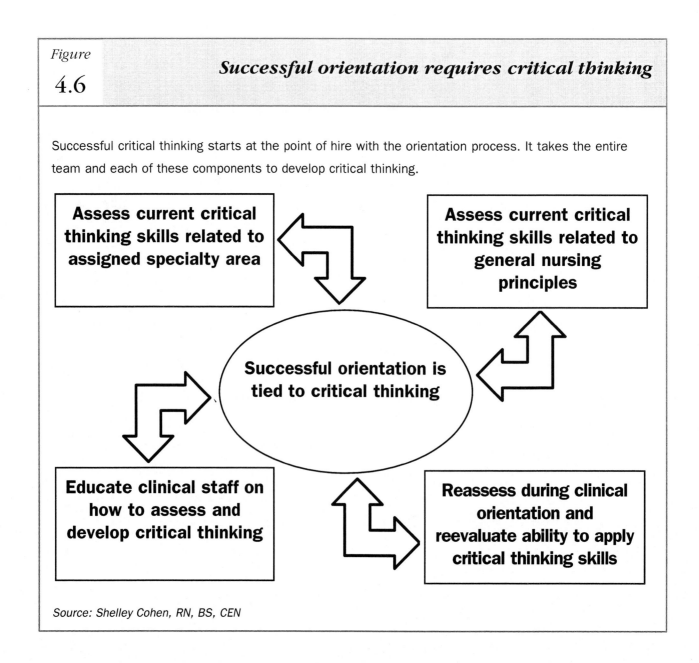

Figure **4.6**

Successful orientation requires critical thinking

Successful critical thinking starts at the point of hire with the orientation process. It takes the entire team and each of these components to develop critical thinking.

Assess current critical thinking skills related to assigned specialty area

Assess current critical thinking skills related to general nursing principles

Successful orientation is tied to critical thinking

Educate clinical staff on how to assess and develop critical thinking

Reassess during clinical orientation and reevaluate ability to apply critical thinking skills

Source: Shelley Cohen, RN, BS, CEN

     Critical Thinking in the Emergency Department

Nursing practice that promotes and motivates critical thinking

Maintaining momentum

Once nurses have finished with orientation, the journey to critical thinking becomes more subtle.

After spending time and money to teach nursing staff about critical thinking skills, you probably have high hopes for seeing these skills translated into improvements in patient care. Yet if you do not create an environment that supports and motivates ongoing development of critical thinking, it is unrealistic to expect most staff to continue to practice it.

Immediately after completing a course on critical thinking, most experienced nurses will independently implement critical thinking in their daily practice. But without a setting that supports the ongoing development and use of these skills, nurses will easily fall back into practice patterns that do not involve a higher level of reasoning. New graduate nurses have no previous experiences or practices to fall back on, but the reality of practice may reduce their ability to think critically. How they are mentored and the role models of experienced nurses around them will determine what they will offer for patient care.

Nurses respond well to challenging work environments and practice settings that embrace critical thinking. Nurses who practice critical thinking operate at a higher level, meaning they are more likely to be stimulated and fulfilled professionally. This may be demonstrated by

- interest in committee involvement
- support for quality improvement efforts
- proactively seeking to attend ongoing education
- initiating more collaborate efforts with other members of the team
- early identification of acute changes in patients

In addition to the preceptor/mentor, the following people and practices play important roles in encouraging the ongoing development and implementation of critical thinking and practice standards. Identify the areas in which you can implement the most immediate change.

- Nurse manager

- Nurse educator

- Defining critical-thinking expectations in a written format through
    - job descriptions
    - clinical guidelines
    - policy and procedure

Nurse managers and staff educators

Newly hired and seasoned staff will look to nurse managers, as the leader of the department(s), to validate how much importance they should place on this "critical thinking stuff." They will look to staff educators to provide leadership and ongoing education.

Nurse managers and staff educators should set expectations for critical thinking by expecting staff to have the ability to

- organize
- prioritize
- delegate
- practice safely
- apply reasoning when making decisions

These are the skills of nurses who have the ability to make appropriate decisions, and they will have been discussed through classroom sessions and during orientation. But if managers and educators do not maintain the momentum through a culture that requires ongoing development of critical thinking, your orientation efforts will fall short. You need to ensure a patient-care environment that nurtures critical thinkers, that stimulates them and motivates them to engage in a discussion in their minds. This discussion is all about one question: *Is this in the best interest of the patient?*

Take out one of your time sheets, and as you look down the list of names, ask yourself how you really feel about each nurse's ability to demonstrate these attributes. Use Figure 5.1 to assist you as you validate educational and remediation needs of individual staff. This tool also may be used by preceptors and senior staff—such as charge nurses—who are involved in assessing staff performance.

Figure 5.1	Critical thinking skills assessment— Nurse manager/staff educator tool														

Staff name	1	2	3	4	5	6	7	8	9	10	11	12	13	14	15

1. Asks pertinent questions
2. Assesses statements/arguments
3. Displays curiosity
4. Listens to others and gives feedback
5. Looks for evidence or proof
6. Examines problems closely
7. Rejects incorrect information
8. Wants to find answers
9. Independently thinks things through
10. Displays confidence about actions
11. Can analyze an argument
12. Looks at the evidence and facts
13. Considers consequences before acting
14. Recognizes contradictions
15. Evaluates policy and considers appropriateness for patient

Source: Shelley Cohen, RN, BS, CEN

Making critical thinking part of the culture

For critical thinking to be a part of your nursing culture, it has to be more than something that is simply "checked off" once a year. The concepts of reasoning should be ingrained in the following:

- job descriptions
- clinical guidelines
- policy and procedure
- performance reviews
- processes that incorporate goal setting

Job descriptions

Job descriptions that do not reflect the reality of what staff members actually do or are expected to do provide no foundation for staff accountability, but it is impossible to include every item, task, or responsibility that nurses will be expected to perform. Therefore, using terminology related to critical thinking sends a clear message that "other duties" may be required.

To improve the content of your job descriptions, consider

- Involving staff in the process of updating and reviewing job descriptions on a regular basis. Ask prompting questions to assist staff in this process:

  - What are you doing on a regular basis that is not on the job description?
  - What is on the job description that you no longer do?
  - What do you feel should be added that will help hold all nurses more accountable?

- Identify patient scenarios that demonstrated a lack of critical thinking:

  - Was there anything absent from the job description that made it difficult to hold staff accountable for their action or lack of action?

- Were there practice standards related to the scenario that were not followed? If so, do the current job descriptions define the expectation that staff members are responsible for maintaining a current knowledge base for the specialty in which they provide nursing care?

Job description examples

Nurses will use critical thinking skills to determine action needed for risk-management concerns such as patient falls, patients refusing care, or visitors with unacceptable behavior.

- The reassessment process for post-sedation patients includes the items below (provide actual process). Nurses are expected to critically think through the needs of each post-sedation patient who may require more frequent reassessments.

- Emergency nurses will use critical thinking skills when determining the triage level in the process of sorting ED patients.

- ED nurses will use critical thinking skills to manage their workload and offer support to the team as needed.

Clinical guidelines

We all know staff members who attend training events and seminars, yet do not have the ability to apply what they learned in the clinical setting. An example of this may be the nurse who successfully passes the ACLS written exam and the testing stations, yet he or she is disorganized and lacks knowledge in an actual resuscitative event. The same principle applies to critical thinking concepts. The nurse may have been taught critical thinking principles, yet when performing patient care he or she does not appear to "have it together." This may present itself as disorganization or even in an actual patient error from a lack of judgment.

Clinical guidelines—also referred to as care paths and clinical pathways—provide evidence-based interventions and direction to set standards of practice for specific patient clinical presentations. These models require the nurse to use reasoning and prioritization to determine when to take each step in the guideline. (If nurses are unable to follow clinical guidelines, they need remediation and further help.)

The implementation of clinical guidelines demonstrates the use of standards of practice, as well as implying that nurses possess the critical thinking needed to apply the guidelines.

Policy and procedure

When relating policy and procedure to critical thinking, you should expect nurses to grasp the following:

- Know where policies and procedures are kept
- Read the policies and procedures
- Understand what each policy is asking/requiring
- Identify the patient/situation for which to engage each policy or procedure

---

Policy and procedure examples

Reassessment of the ED patient

The ED nurse will use critical thinking skills in determining what aspect of the patient's presentation requires reassessment, and how often this should occur and be documented.

Patient visitors in the ED

The ED charge nurse will employ critical thinking to identify those situations that may require an exception to the visitor policy. These scenarios may include a patient death or impending death, a victim of abuse/neglect, a family member also ill or injured, etc.

Performance reviews

The annual review is an opportunity for the manager to reinforce expectations regarding critical thinking with each member of the nursing staff. Again, Figure 5.1 (page 76) can be used or adapted to outline areas of strength and weakness for each nurse. You also may want to have the nursing staff perform a self-assessment of their ability to think critically prior to the annual review. Figure 5.2 is an example of a self-assessment tool.

Figure 5.2	Annual performance review— Self-assessment of critical thinking

Employee name: _____ **Date of self-assessment:** _____

Please rate your ability to apply critical thinking in the following areas:

5 = I always do this
4 = I do this most of the time
3 = I sometimes do this
2 = I rarely do this and realize I need to be more aware in this area
1 = I never do this and realize I need some help to improve on this

1.	I ask pertinent questions.	5	4	3	2	1
2.	I assess statements/arguments before making decisions.	5	4	3	2	1
3.	I am always curious about things and want to learn.	5	4	3	2	1
4.	I listen to others and give feedback.	5	4	3	2	1
5.	I look for evidence or proof before doing what someone else says I should do.	5	4	3	2	1
6.	I examine problems closely.	5	4	3	2	1
7.	I know when information is incorrect and I reject it.	5	4	3	2	1
8.	I want to find answers.	5	4	3	2	1
9.	I independently think things through.	5	4	3	2	1
10.	I am confident in my actions.	5	4	3	2	1
11.	I can analyze an argument..	5	4	3	2	1
12.	I look at the evidence and facts.	5	4	3	2	1
13.	I consider consequences before acting.	5	4	3	2	1
14.	I recognize contradictions.	5	4	3	2	1
15.	I evaluate policy and consider its appropriateness for the patient.	5	4	3	2	1

Source: Shelley Cohen, RN, BS, CEN

This self-assessment tool can be compared to the worksheet you prepared for the employee's performance review and the employee's goals for the coming year (Figure 5.3 can be used to plan short- and long-term goals), and can be specific to discuss judgment and reasoning when appropriate. Other benefits of staff performing a self-assessment of their abilities are

- it details specific expectations from both you and the patient

- in the process of completing the tool, questions should and will arise regarding critical-thinking concepts, prompting further discussion

- it requires them to consider specific patient scenarios when they have actually displayed these abilities

Figure	**Goals worksheet**
5.3	

Name: _____

Job title: _____

Today's date: _____

Short-term goals

In the next year, I would like to do the following:

Add _____ to my job description

Take _____ continuing education classes

Work on projects related to improving _____

Long-term goals

In the next 2–5 years I would like to do the following:

Have completed _____

Make these changes in my job _____

Have accomplished _____

Obtain certification in _____

Source: Shelley Cohen, RN, BS, CEN

As you and the nurse identify areas that need improvement, first prompt the nurse to offer suggestions and resources before you do. Remember, part of your role is to coach staff—if you provide all the answers all the time, you are stifling their critical thinking.

Goal setting

When staff demonstrate unacceptable behavior or unsafe patient practices, take the opportunity to discuss the importance of critical thinking. From point of hire to annual review to daily patient care, judgment will always play a central role. When setting new goals in response to unacceptable behavior or unsafe patient events, relate the goals to the nurse developing better judgment and displaying higher levels of critical thinking.

Figure 5.4 contains examples of what to consider saying and how to document the conversation and conclusions reached.

Figure 5.4	Setting goals for improvement

Should Nancy present to the department late on another shift between today's date and _____ she will know that

- an off-going shift member will be delayed
- an oncoming shift nurse will have to take an additional assignment
- patient care will be directly affected

Nancy has the ability to critically think through the ramifications for when staff do not present on time for their shift and she has outlined these in our meeting today.

Timothy is aware of the resources available to nurses in the department when they are in need of detailed medication information. He agrees that if he had looked up the information on _____ and applied nursing judgment, the patient would not have been given the dose.

Timothy will demonstrate appropriate nursing judgment when administering medication by

- using available resources in the department such as reference books by or calling the pharmacy.

- successfully completing a written medication assessment tool, achieving a grade of 90% or better. This will be done within the next 15 days.

- having the charge nurse check all calculations for pediatric medications for the next 30 days.

Source: Shelley Cohen, RN, BS, CEN

Chapter 6

Novice to expert: Setting realistic expectations for critical thinking

LEARNING OBJECTIVE

After reading this section, the participant should be able to

• evaluate the challenges facing new and experienced nurses in incorporating critical thinking skills into practice and strategies to help meet expectations

Setting realistic expectations

As you approach and consider methods not only to teach but also to motivate critical thinking, it is essential that your expectations meet the abilities of the nurse. The last thing you want is an environment that creates fear of critical-thinking expectations. We want staff to embrace the concept, confident in their abilities to develop their thinking and reasoning skills.

Align your expectations more with what it is realistic to expect from nurses, rather than what you hope they can do. As you set your expectations, consider each nurse's potential, opportunities to perform, opportunities to reach goals, and the outcomes you hope each nurse will achieve.

Make sure your expectations are

- realistic
- supported with appropriate tools and resources
- appropriate for the specialty area in which the nurse works
- flexible to meet a variety of learning needs
- clarified in writing
- related to the performance review

Novice to competent: New graduate nurses

It may seem obvious that the expectations for critical thinking displayed by new graduate nurses would not be the same as those for experienced nurses. Yet many new graduate nurses are facing peer groups who have already decided what they should/should not know. Preceptors, nurse educators, and nurse managers are the ones who must set the expectations for new graduates, not the experienced nurses on the unit. Preceptors, nurse educators, and nurse managers should be the ones who communicate the expectations for new graduates to the rest of the staff.

When new graduate nurses join the emergency department, use the opportunity for the team to consider the experience of new nurses and what new graduates have to cope with. Include the following points in the discussion to enlighten staff and help them have a better understanding of why the expectations on new graduates are different today than they were in previous decades:

- Many students today have fewer clinical opportunities than most current nurses had in school.

- Students today have to contend with a chronic shortage of nursing faculty across the country.

- Many nursing schools "teach to the boards" and great focus is placed on successful completion of the NCLEX.

- Students' limited clinical time may not have exposed them to challenging patients similar to those seen in your environment.

- In years past, nurses gained several years of experience before becoming specialty nurses. Now many enter a specialty straight out of school.

Let it be known that you will not tolerate staff members who are unwilling to accept today's realities for new graduates. Do not allow statements such as, "Back in my day we were expected to . . . " The manager, preceptor, and educator need to promptly address individuals who make such comments so the message is clear: This is unacceptable behavior. Work together to script appropriate responses that hold those individuals accountable, such as, "We are not practicing 1962 nursing care here. Are you?"

As new graduates move further along and out of their orientation period, assist in the transition from novice staff nurse to competent staff nurse by considering the following:

- Use tools that allow new graduates to self-assess their level of critical thinking

- Reevaluate decision-making skills throughout the orientation process

- Promptly clarify all questions regarding expectations

- Promote a culture and environment that encourage critical thinking

- Remember that critical thinking is a process that develops and grows throughout the career

- Bear in mind that new graduates who do not employ critical thinking in their personal lives will face the greatest challenges in incorporating it into their nursing care

Greatest challenges for new graduate nurses

Among the many challenges new graduates will face—and obstacles to the development of their critical thinking—are the patients in their care who have bad outcomes and the providers who are unwilling to collaborate with them. The first makes them ask the question, "What should I have done?" The second makes them unwilling to use their critical thinking skills, because they feel they are not needed.

The first year after graduation is a time for education, and care must be taken that new graduates are not frightened to make a decision or feel constantly indecisive in the care they provide.

Coaching new graduates through bad patient outcomes

- Allow them to grieve through their error or omission. Whether patients are in their care for one hour or one week, in their minds, they are still "my patient."

- As nurses we tend to beat ourselves up when we make a medication or other error. After we are done whipping ourselves, we move on. New graduate nurses need time to go through a process where they review what happened and how they would approach it differently next time. Our job is to coach them away from the blame and move them toward learning experiences.

- Provide them with more than one opportunity to sit with a supportive mentor or preceptor to review the scenario that led to the patient outcome.

- Make sure you are the person who debriefs the nurses. Don't expose them to the nurse who says, "I told you this would happen if you let new grads in here."

- Even if the bad outcome was not related to something they did or did not do, they still may feel like it was their fault. Coach them that a guilt trip will not change the outcome of the scenario.

- If they are not willing to take responsibility or accountability for something they did or did not do for the patient, recognize this as a patient safety warning. These nurses will require further assessment of their critical-thinking capabilities and ongoing involvement with the nurse manager.

Growing collaborative relationships with the medical staff

Working with the medical staff can be intimidating for new graduates if steps are not taken to develop relationships. Simple steps can help promote the new relationship and build a basis of good feeling so that both sides may build trust.

- Have someone introduce new graduates to the medical staff as they arrive on the unit.

- If medical staff members have had previous negative experiences with new graduate nurses, make time to discuss the critical-thinking training you are providing these new graduates.

- Circulate a memo to the medical staff introducing the new graduates and briefly outlining expectations, the critical thinking training, and names of the preceptors.

- Ask the members of the medical staff to think back to their own internships and remind them that critical thinking will develop with their support.

- If the new graduates are in a specialty area, see if they can spend some shifts in the offices of those specialties where they can observe and work alongside the practitioner.

- In your critical-thinking training, include scenarios that allow novice nurses to explore options for how to respond to challenging times and conversations with providers. This is part of teaching them how to respond professionally to any challenge in the health-care environment.

Growing collaborative relationships with the interdisciplinary team

New graduates also face expectations from other team members, which may include ancillary services such as radiology, respiratory therapy, laboratory, and pharmacy. Build a pattern of success for new graduates nurse by communicating with other services:

- Dates of new graduates' arrivals and the departments/areas to which they are assigned

- Include time for new nurses to partner with other services

- Discuss the time frame of the orientation process and give a list of realistic expectations related to their services

- Incorporate interdisciplinary team members' skills and experiences as part of the new graduate's education by including them as faculty for classroom time

When new graduates fail to reach competent levels of critical thinking

For managers and preceptors, one of the greatest challenges is when you are confronted with newly graduated nurses who just don't seem to "get it." There will be times, despite your best efforts and resources, when the concept of critical thinking will not be grasped in a realistic time frame. This situation must be addressed promptly to be fair to the newly hired nurse, the preceptor, the staff, and, of course, the patients.

While it's important to understand the emotional elements involved for new graduate nurses, this does not change the fact that the level of nursing practice being displayed is unsafe and unacceptable. It is misleading to allow the new graduate to carry on believing that "things will just work out."

Key steps to take when new graduates are not progressing with critical thinking development include:

- Identifying early on those new graduates who are not meeting expectations

- Defining which expectations they are not meeting and providing examples

 Critical Thinking in the Emergency Department

- Offering and providing remediation with new expectations and a written timeline for meeting the expectations

- If remediation does not change nursing practice, the manager should meet with human resources to determine the next appropriate step

For new graduates who continue to fail to progress, consider options such as these:

- Transferring the nurse, depending on his or her weaknesses, to a department outside of the ED that has

  - less-complex patients
  - fewer multitasking skills needed
  - fewer unplanned scenarios
  - lower patient-assignment loads

- Extending the probationary period

- Collaborating with faculty from his or her school of nursing for mediation direction

In all of this, do not disregard your obligations to patients and the State Board of Nursing as they relate to patient safety.

Competent to expert: Experienced nurses

Many of the principles that relate to new graduate nurses also apply to those with more experience. One of the challenges with experienced nurses is that many in the peer group have higher expectations and often believe these expectations are being met, even if they have no evidence to show this. For example, they see the experienced nurse demonstrate a particular skill or task well, and then assume all the nurse's skills are at that level. This type of assumption can be dangerous, and can mean experienced nurses receive less support and training for them to develop their critical thinking skills.

Once again, it is important to define realistic expectations for all newly hired nursing staff and establish timelines for when they should accomplish these expectations.

When experienced nurses join your unit, remind the team of the following concepts:

- Just because someone successfully completes an ACLS course does not mean they can function in a cardiopulmonary-arrest situation

- If team members do not share concerns related to new nurse performance with the preceptor, educator, or manager, then issues cannot be addressed

- Doing a procedure faster does not imply you understand why you are doing it

- People can "talk" a great story; the test is whether they can perform at that level

- If staff nurses don't get involved in the process of orienting newly hired nurses, we cannot truly assess their abilities to think critically and act critically

In addition to experienced nurses who have just joined the unit, you should also assess and support the critical thinking development of nurses who have long been there.

Use assessment tools such as Figures 4.1, 4.2 and 5.2 to validate the ability of experienced nurses to apply critical thinking in their practice settings. For those who are unable to demonstrate their ability, initiate a remediation process in conjunction with the nurse manager.

Handling experienced nurses who need remediation

When you are confronted with seasoned nurses who are unable to meet your expectations, consider the following:

- If a new hire, do they need a different preceptor?
- If a new hire, are they still in their probationary period?
- Is there one area in which they are unable to attain a skill, or is it an overall care issue?
- If they have been staff members for a while, how has this been handled in the past?

Novice to expert: Setting realistic expectations for critical thinking

Your facility needs to use consistency when addressing this sensitive issue. If nurses are long past the orientation period and are not meeting critical-thinking expectations, find out how this has been handled with other nurses in the past. You may want to set a new precedent for how it will be handled in the future.

Because the ability to think critically is one that is ongoing and constantly being developed, it requires ongoing reevaluation. For example, just because the nurse you hired four years ago demonstrated good strategies in nursing care when he or she was hired, does not mean he or she still practices within those same principles. Consider these elements that occur in your patient care areas:

- New procedures
- New evidence and research that demonstrates a different approach to particular diagnoses
- The multitude of new medications added to the formulary each year
- New standards of practice from regulatory agencies and authorities

With this list in mind, and considering that healthcare is in constant flux, it makes sense to design a process to continually reassess nurses' ability to think critically. You can directly involve staff in this process by

- incorporating critical-thinking language and expectations in written documents such as

  - policies and procedures
  - employee handbook
  - clinical pathways/guidelines
  - job descriptions
  - performance reviews

- having staff review these written expectations annually and offer suggestions for change

- having staff complete self-assessment sheets (see Figures 4.1, 4.2 and 5.2)

- requiring staff to present examples of how they have displayed critical thinking in their patient care at their performance reviews

Measuring critical thinking in daily practice

How do you know whether nurses are thinking critically in their practice? Regardless of their level of experience, once they have completed orientation and have been "checked off" you are implying they no longer need daily precepting. You are making a statement that they have demonstrated the ability to meet their job description. If you do not feel they can perform their job description/requirements independently, then the orientation process needs to be extended.

Demonstrating they can think critically is more than being checked off on being able to perform a task or procedure. Use and adapt the sample tools throughout the book—such as Figure 4.4, which assesses their ability to think through what patients are telling them—to evaluate their level of performance. Using standard criteria for the evaluation will help you validate whether critical thinking is part of their nursing practice, for both experienced and inexperienced nurses.

Examples of demonstrating critical thinking

Emergency room nurses demonstrate critical thinking by

- identifying early symptoms of shock
- asking every patient safety questions at each visit to identify victims of violence
- evaluating the intake and output of an admitted patient being held over in the ED
- asking the provider if he or she noticed the wound on the patient's posterior thorax
- discussing with EMS about the living conditions in which the patient was found
- recognizing that a patient with a cough, who is also an inmate, is a high-risk patient for TB

Applying critical thinking to nursing documentation

Turning critical thinking into critical writing

Critical writing is as important as critical thinking. Good documentation is a vital part of patient care and nurses need to be able to validate in the written medical record what they did or what they chose not to do. We think of the medical record as a storybook that tells what happened to the patient from the point of entry into the healthcare system to the point of exit from the system. With all of today's risk management and legal concerns that challenge healthcare delivery systems as well as the caregivers, it is vital to demonstrate steps and actions taken to support the patient.

Identifying a patient problem, potential consequences, and necessary actions are vital elements of critical thinking for nurses. However, without appropriate and timely documentation, there is no written record of what has occurred.

Transforming critical thinking into the written format provides

- a legal record to support a nurse's

    - identification of a problem
    - actions taken in response to the problem
    - patient outcomes related to any intervention
    - collaboration with other members of the healthcare team
    - compliance with nursing standards of practice

- a timetable of the events to reference as a tool in determining ongoing care and needs of the patient

- validation of the nursing process that incorporated critical thinking

 Critical Thinking in the Emergency Department

> Figure
> 7.1
>
> *Eight common charting errors*
>
> ---
>
> Accurate and complete nursing documentation is essential for demonstrating compliance with standards, delivery of state-of-the-art nursing care, and the ability to communicate effectively with everyone involved in patient care. Therefore, it is important to recognize common charting mistakes and ways to educate your staff about them.
>
> Charting mistakes can lead to allegations of negligence. The following list describes the eight most common charting mistakes, along with how and why you should avoid them.
>
> ### 1. Failure to document pertinent health or drug information
>
> Nurses conducting admission assessments are responsible for acquiring all pertinent health data that will influence the plan of care. As silly as this mistake may seem, nursing admission assessments and transfer notes are often left incomplete.
>
> Good history-taking skills are especially important during the initial admission assessment, as the assessment is important to the safety and well-being of the patient. Any health information that is not gathered when taking the history or not documented in the appropriate location on the clinical record can lead to adverse consequences.
>
> To avoid this kind of mistake, ensure that your staff members know how to take thorough histories and focus particularly on patients who cannot communicate effectively, are poor historians, or have dementia. Remind staff members to document conversations with significant others, the transferring agency, or any other source of information. Provide them with continuing education regarding communication skills needed to ascertain a complete and thorough patient history.
>
> Also ensure that any important health or medication information is documented and communicated to others effectively. Neglecting to communicate an important piece of patient information can leave a nurse open to allegations of negligence. To avoid this, record the information in all of the locations designated by your policies. Also, encourage the use of bright labels and other accepted means of communicating the information.

Figure

7.1

Eight common charting errors (cont.)

---

2. Failure to record nursing actions

There needs to be a way to communicate every nursing action, and nurses must get into the habit of documenting them as close as possible to the time they occur. Unfortunately, charting is often left to the end of many nurses' busy days. This is not a good habit, but often difficult to break. Here are some guidelines to follow:

- Record all observations, assessments, and actions on the flow sheet or designated form.

- You must chart as close to the time as possible, even if it is a one- or two-line entry.

- Reduce redundancy and only chart the fact once. You do not need to repeat the same data in more than one place. Just be sure it can be found in the clinical record. If there is redundancy in your documentation system, revise it.

3. Failure to record medications given

This may seem obvious, but how many times have you reviewed a medication administration record (MAR) and found that the previous shift's nurse said in his or her report that the patient had been medicated even though you could not find it documented in the medical record?

Avoid nursing negligence by recording all medications given and the rationale for those not given, even if you may perceive them as insignificant. Always investigate when you suspect that a medication may have been administered but not recorded.

4. Recording on the wrong chart

Sometimes, a simple mistake of misfiling can lead a nurse to chart on the wrong patient. Staff are especially vulnerable to this error when patients with similar names are on the same unit, so you need a system of identification that is clear and as foolproof as possible.

Figure

7.1

Figure

7.1

Eight common charting errors (cont.)

Errors in this category include

- transcribing medication orders onto the wrong patient's chart.

- writing progress notes without confirming the accuracy of the chart you chose. To prevent this error, look at the external name on the chart and always look at the name stamped at the top of the document.

Whenever possible, do not assign the same nurse to patients with the same name. And always ensure compliance with the National Patient Safety Goal that refers to proper patient identification prior to procedures and medication administration.

5. Failure to document a discontinued medication

Nurses are responsible for ensuring safe patient care at all levels. When a medication has been ordered to be discontinued, the change must be appropriately noted according to policy and communicated to the next shift's nurse. Nurses also need to comply with the organization's policies concerning cross-checking the physician orders with the MAR. Doing so can prevent serious complications.

6. Failure to document drug reactions/changes in patient's condition

The literature on "failure to rescue" points to this potential error. Nurses are responsible for the assessment of a patient's reaction to medication and for the identification of any change in a patient's condition. They must have the skill and knowledge to anticipate the clinical needs of a patient. They must also possess critical thinking skills to intervene appropriately in any adverse reaction or worsening of the patient's condition. But performing this assessment, identification, and intervention is not enough. Nurses must also document that they have done so.

| Figure 7.1 | *Eight common charting errors (cont.)* |

7. Improper transcription of orders or transcription of improper orders

The registered nurse can be held liable for transcribing improper doses that led to a patient's injury. The nurse can also be held liable for transcribing and carrying out an order they know to be inaccurate or suspect to be incorrect.

If the nurses discuss both the order and their concerns with physicians, they must document these conversations. In addition, if nurses still maintain that administration of the medication or proceeding with a procedure is not in the best interest of the patient, they must activate the chain of command and document that as well.

In contemporary nursing practice, all nurses must know medications or research a new medication prior to administration. If a nurse is not familiar with a procedure and does not seek supervision or assistance with it, questions of clinical competence and ensuring patient safety will come into play if there is any question of malpractice. The public expects that we will continue to keep our professional skills and knowledge up to date. Falling short of this will put a nurse in a difficult position from which to defend her- or himself.

8. Writing illegible or incomplete records

Illegible handwriting is no longer tolerated by regulatory and accreditation surveyors. With the goal of improving patient safety, the days of laughing at someone's handwriting are over. All providers who document in the clinical record must ensure that what they have written is readable. Should the clinical record be reviewed, it is essential that the author of the record be able to clearly read it. Some hospitals have instituted illegible handwriting policies to improve compliance with legible-documentation standards and to improve patient safety.

Source: DuClos-Miller, P. 2004. Managing Documentation Risk: A Guide for Nurse Managers. *Marblehead, MA: HCPro, Inc.*

Examples of critical writing skills

The following are examples of the application of critical writing skills in patient documentation.

Patient case 1

1019	Responding to patient call light, I found patient on floor beside bed, unresponsive and pulseless.
	Both side rails were in place and locked. Room panic button pulled and Code Blue called; CPR initiated.
	Refer to code flow sheet for code details.
1036	Patient transferred to ICU via stretcher with Dr. Jones and ICU staff.
1042	Per request of Dr. Jones, I notified patient's family by phone and they are en route to the hospital.

Documentation demonstrates the nurse continued to use critical thinking once patient care was transferred to the ICU staff. Critical thinking and documentation may be related to the family or caregiver, not just the patient.

Patient case 2

1036	In patient's room for IV start and prep for surgery. When I inquired if patient had any questions, she cried. Patient states, "I don't understand why they need to take out my ovaries--I am only 25 years old." I suggested she speak to her doctor prior to receiving anesthesia.
1045	Dr. McCall paged and informed of patient's concerns. He will be in to see her before anesthesia is initiated.
1050	I spoke with S. Kyle, Nurse Anesthetist, and updated him on need to hold anesthesia until patient speaks with Dr. McCall. "Alert" sticker placed on front of patient chart.

Documentation reflects nurse's use of critical thinking in recognizing that it was important for anesthesia to be directly told of the patient's need to speak with her physician while still able to understand need for and expected results from her planned surgery. Documenting that the "alert" sticker was placed on the chart shows the nurse also critically thought through that other members of the team needed this information as well.

Patient case 3

250	Patient states, "I fell out of my deer stand when I went hunting yesterday."
	Presents ambulatory complaining of right ankle pain, walks with limp.
	Patient immediately placed in spine precautions due to mechanism of injury.

Documentation shows evidence that the nurse used critical thinking to suspect more than an ankle injury due to the mechanism of how the patient was injured. Should the patient have a spine injury, there is validation to show that it was considered and addressed by the triage nurse.

Patient case 4

1008	Patient noted to be short of breath and diaphoretic.
1009	Physician and respiratory therapy paged from patient room.
1012	Oxygen at 10 liters via non-rebreather mask.
1016	Skin warm and dry, color pink, mental status alert and oriented.
1021	Dr. Jones at bedside.

Time elements demonstrate that priorities were initiated in the appropriate order.

Patient case 5

2207	Pain medication given as ordered.
2228	Patient has no relief of pain and states, "It is worse than before."
	Right leg is pink and warm to the touch, cap refill to toes is 3 seconds.
	Patient has no change in sensation from original assessment at 2100.
	Dr. Benington notified.
2245	Dr. Benington at bedside.

Documentation demonstrates multiple simultaneous actions to meet unexpected needs of patient. Patient's response or lack of response is identified, and the appropriate interventions are then noted. This demonstrates the nurse used critical thinking to relate the change in pain as an early sign of compartment syndrome.

Patient case 6

0310	In responding to patient's call light, patient states, "You people are really stupid. I want to speak with someone in charge right now." I explained to patient that I would page the house supervisor, Mr. Bentley, who would be happy to come and speak with him.
0311	Security notified per policy relating to potential for violence.
0315	Mr. Bentley at bedside of patient who is pacing in room and using profanity in a loud voice. Patient is requesting to sign out of hospital. I called Dr. Wright and informed him of the situation. Call transferred to patient's phone per Dr. Wright.
	Patient threw phone at Mr. Bentley; security outside room secured environment.
	Sheriff's department contacted via red phone.

Documentation relates events related to potential or actual violence/harm to patient or others. Demonstrates application of department procedures, and risk potential for other patients and staff.

Relating critical thinking to its higher purpose

In nursing, we tend to work toward achieving goals as the end of a process, when many times meeting the goal is just the beginning. In this book, Polly Gerber Zimmermann reminds us that *learning to think critically is a journey, not a destination.* The foundation of critical thinking skills you build for nurses will be directly reflected in your ability to continue on this path. The ability to meet the needs of our patients is a moving walkway that seems to go on forever. Each specialty of healthcare delivery is faced with having to provide care to more patients at a faster pace with fewer resources.

Whether you work in acute care, rehab, home health, or medical-office settings, or in any other environment, nurses are the people patients and families turn to. They turn to us for clarification, guidance, hope, and the truth.

While driving home from the hospital, I was listening to a postal worker in New Orleans being interviewed on public radio. The postal worker was delivering mail to a district recently reopened after Hurricane Katrina. The interview went along these lines:

Q: What kind of challenges are you facing with this delivery area?
A: Well, there are lots of challenges, such as the debris and trash.

Q: Is it difficult to tell whether or not it is the right house you are delivering to?
*A: If the number is no longer there or the mailbox is gone we are supposed to use **deductive reasoning** to determine if it is the right house. For example, I might look to see if it is a consecutive number.*

This interview reminds us that we use critical thinking in our daily lives without realizing it. For example we think critically

- at the grocery store to determine if the sale price is really a sale or just a cheaper price on a smaller container

- when our child tells us, "I did study for that exam," yet you never saw a book in his or her room

- at the dentist office when we decide whether to pay to fix the tooth or have it pulled

We cannot continue to improve the quality of care we deliver without engaging our reasoning. The ability to reason and consider actions or inactions is a feature of critical thinking that provides a safe patient-care environment. Recognizing the best interest of the patient is paramount in quality-improvement processes. As you consider all of the efforts in which your organization is engaged regarding meeting regulatory standards remember this:

Staff members cannot meet the needs of patients if they cannot recognize those needs.

Chapter 9

Resources and tools

This chapter contains additional tools and resources to assist you in assessing and developing ED nurses' critical thinking capabilities at the point of hire, during orientation, and through ongoing development and review. This chapter contains

- a list of further reading and resources

- additional sample questions

- Figure 9.1, which is a handout that can be given to attendees of a critical thinking class who want further information and study materials

- Figure 9.2, which contains unfolding teaching scenarios that can be used for discussing critical thinking

- Figure 9.3, which contains examples of teachable moments

- Figure 9.4, which is a teaching tool about critical thinking skills related to geriatric patients

- Figure 9.5, which is a sample critical thinking–skills class agenda that can be customized for any facility

- Figures 9.6–9.10, which are worksheets that can be used or adapted for critical thinking classes, during orientation, or for ongoing critical thinking development

Resources and further reading

Publications

Emergency Nurses Association. *Orientation to Emergency Nursing*, 2nd ed. Available from *www.ena.org*.

Emergency Nurses Association. 1999. *Standards of Emergency Nursing Practice*, 4th ed.

Bemis, Patricia Ann. 2005. *Emergency Nursing Bible*, 3rd ed. Rocklidge, FL: National Nurses in Business Association.

Cohen, Shelley. 2002. *101 Triage Tips*. Hohenwald, TN: Health Resources Unlimited.

Doan-Johnson, S., and A. Woods, eds. 2005. *Nursing Made Incredibly Easy*. Philadelphia: Lippincott Williams & Wilkins.

DuClos-Miller, P. 2004. *Managing Documentation Risk: A Guide for Nurse Managers*. Marblehead, MA: HCPro.

Grossman, Valerie. 2003. *Quick Reference to Triage*. Philadelphia: Lippincott Williams & Wilkins.

Lee, N. Genell. 2001. *Legal Concepts and Issues in Emergency Care*. St. Louis: Saunders.

Lipe, S. K. and S. Beasley. 2004. *Critical Thinking in Nursing: A Cognitive Skills Workbook*. Philadelphia: Lippincott Williams & Wilkins.

Proehl, Jean A. 2004. *Emergency Nursing Procedures*, 3rd ed. St. Louis: Saunders.

Rubenfeld, M. G., and B. K. Scheffer. 2006. *Critical Thinking Tactics for Nurses*. Sudbury, MA: Jones and Bartlett.

Springhouse. 2004. *Nurses Legal Handbook*. Philadelphia: Lippincott Williams & Wilkins.

Springhouse. 2006. *Professional Guide to Signs & Symptoms*, 5th ed. Philadelphia: Lippincott Williams & Wilkins.

Wright, Donna. 1998. *The Ultimate Guide to Competency Assessment in Healthcare*. Eau Claire, WI: PESI Healthcare.

Yocum, Fay. 1999. *Documentation Skills for Quality Patient Care*. Dayton, OH: Awareness Productions.

Zimmermann, Polly Gerber, and Robert D. Herr. 2005. *Triage Nursing Secrets*. St. Louis: Mosby.

Web sites

Health Resources Unlimited: *www.hru.net*
- Triage tips, risk management tips

Emergency Nurses Association: *www.ena.org*
- Multiple resources including document sharing

Emergency Nursing World: *www.enw.org*
- Multiple resources including document sharing

EMedHome.com: *www.emedhome.com*
- Clinical pearls, case studies

American College of Emergency Physicians: *www.acep.org*
- Position statements, cases

The Sullivan Group Law Firm: *www.thesullivangroup.com*
- Newsletter reviewing ED cases

National Center for Emergency Medicine Informatics: *www.ncemi.org*
- Clinical cases and challenges

Enchanted Learning: *www.enchantedlearning.com*
  - Anatomy diagrams/glossaries and more

North Central Regional Educational Laboratory (NCREL®): *www.ncrel.org*
  - Resources defining critical thinking

The Advisory Board Company: *www.advisory.com*
  - Multiple resources: Search under new graduate nurse

National Council of State Boards of Nursing: *www.ncsbn.org*
  - Access to all state Boards of Nursing rules and regulations

Additional sample questions

Source: Polly Gerber Zimmermann, RN, MS, MBA, CEN

These questions may be used either for discussion or for a test. Remove answers before providing them to learners. (File can be found under "Additional sample questions" on the accompanying CD-ROM.)

Question: The night nurse walks in to find the patient lying motionless on the floor. List the order that the nurse should complete the following actions.

(Note: This is the new-style sequential NCLEX question. No partial credit is allowed.)

  a. Call the doctor
  b. Write an incident report
  c. Ask the patient what hurts
  d. Place the patient in the bed
  e. Ask the patient why he or she got up
  f. Assess the pulse

Answer: F, C, D, E, A, B

First, establish if the patient is conscious. Is this syncope from a dysrhythmia? Then establish if the patient hit his or her head, rule out neck injury and need for immobilization. Review procedure if that was the case. Could institute a discussion about what patient medications would increase the nurse's concern (warfarin/Coumadin). Then move the patient.

Discuss how often we see people do E first, but does it really matter? After immediate needs, ask: What is a common reason for falling? Going to the bathroom.

Question: A 96-year-old patient who was admitted with pneumonia is found crawling out of the bed. What should the nurse do first?

a. Assess the patient's pain level

b. Obtain a pulse oximeter reading

c. Reorient the patient and reinforce the need to stay in bed

d. Apply a Posey jacket

Answer: B

New-onset confusion should have hypoglycemia and inadequate oxygenation ruled out first. The elderly who have decreased respiratory reserve are more prone to complications and atypical presentations.

Follow-up discussion could include how you would handle a low reading, and what else to consider if it was "normal." (How would you expect the result to be different if the patient had COPD?)

One of the most common symptoms for urinary tract infection in patients with Alzheimer's disease is new-onset restlessness.

Could also have a discussion about other considerations: sun-downing, alternatives to restraints, etc.

Consider offering a true "war story" as an accompaniment: Elderly patient kept crawling out of bed. Nurse obtained order and restrained patient. Other nurse took pulse oximetry and found it was 88%.

Use this as a good opportunity to review hospital's restraint policy.

Question: After morning report at 7 a.m., which problem should the nurse take care of first?

    a. Patient going to surgery at 9 a.m. does not have a signed consent

    b. Two-day postop patient has pain at "8"

    c. Pump transfusing blood is beeping "occluded"

    d. Morning temp on one-day postop patient is 100.4°F (38°C)

Answer: C

High-risk procedure: You only have four hours once the blood is on the floor. You need to assess if the patient is bending the arm, kinking the tubing, etc., or if the IV needs to be reassessed.

B (a disability need) would be next.

A can be done later.

D could be atelexasis. Perform an assessment and encourage deep breathing.

Ask what else they need to know about "D"—is this patient immunosuppressed?

Question: The nurse receives the following lab values on the newly admitted client. Which value should the nurse deal with first?

(Note: This is the new-style fill-in-the blank NCLEX question. Also note: AST and ALT were formerly known as SGOT and SGPT.)

Test	Patient result	Normal range
Glucose	193 mg/dL	70–110 mg/dL
BUN	8 mg/dL	10–20 mg/dL
Cr	0.7 mg/dL	0.7–1.2 mg/dL
Sodium	131 mEq/dL	135–145 mEq/dL
Potassium	3.2 mEq/dL	3.5–5.0 mEq/dL
SGOT	1932 IU/L	13–40 IU/L
SGPT	2360 IU/L	7–60 IU/L
Bilirubin total	2.9 mg/dL	0.2–1.2 mg/dL

Answer: Potassium

Potassium is an intracellular electrolyte and a drop of 0.1mEq actually represents a drop of 200mEq. Since potassium affects muscle, the nurse would be most worried about the effect on cardiac muscle.

Sodium is an extracellular electrolyte, so the results are an actual reflection of the current body supply. In addition, the kidney can conserve sodium, but not potassium.

The elevated glucose could be, in part, due to the acute illness. A further workup or insulin could be done later.

The client does have liver enzyme elevation but that is not the priority. It would be a factor in drug dosing.

How will this client appear? Jaundiced.

Question: The nurse receives the following laboratory results for a patient. What is the best interpretation?

Test	Patient result	Normal range
WBC	4.1 K/cmm	4.5–10.0 K/cmm
RBC	3.2 mil/cmm	4.3–5.8 mil/cmm
HGB	11.3 gm/dL	12–15 gm/dL
HCT	29.1%	36–47%
Segs	28%	36–71%
Bands	2%	0–7%
Lymphs	62%	20–40%
Eosinophils	3%	1–6%

a. The patient is immunosuppressed

b. The patient is having an allergic reaction

c. The patient has an acute bacterial infection

d. The patient has a viral infection

Answer: D

Lymphs go up in a viral infection. Depressed, rather than elevated, WBC are more likely with viral. Immunosuppression would result in significant depression of all views. The borderline hemoglobin can also be a result of this. Eosinophils are elevated in an allergic reaction. An acute bacterial infection would typically have an elevated WBC and neutrophils, bands/segs/immature cells.

Question: It is most important for the nurse to care for which new patient complaint first?

    a. Type II DM with a.m. blood sugar of 160mg

    b. Client receiving a K+ rider (IVPB) complaining that the arm is sore

    c. Asthmatic on steroids is catching the flu, temperature 100.4°F (38°C)

    d. Patient with pneumonia's WBC is 15,000 with an elevation in neutrophils

Answer: C

Rule out septic response in an immunosuppressed patient with compromised respiratory function. Then A can be taken care of.

B is an expected complaint. What can the nurse do? It might be possible to slow the infusion rate or further dilute the concentration.

D is an expected finding. What else does the nurse want to know? Patient's temperature and the trend of the WBC: higher, lower, the same. Also verify the patient is on an appropriate antibiotic.

Critical Thinking in the Emergency Department

Figure

9.1

Critical thinking skills course—
Additional resources handout

■ **Dorothy Del Bueno's article about critical thinking displayed by nurses:**

Del Bueno, D. 2001. "Buyer beware: The cost of competence." *Nursing Economics*
19 (6): 259–257.

■ **American Association of Critical-Care Nursing (AACN) decision tree for delegation**
decisions: Available from 101 Columbia, Alisa Viejo, CA 92656-1491; 800/899-2226

■ **Give new graduates "rules" for "telling somebody" by using the criteria developed for**
Rapid Response Team Activation (a concept introduced by the Institute for Healthcare
Improvement [IHI] as part of the "100,000 Lives Campaign.")

- IHI recommendations: *www.ihi.org/IHI/Programs/TransformingCareattheBedside*.

- Scholle, C. C., and C. Mininni. 2006 "Best-practice interventions: How a Rapid Response
  Team saves lives." *Nursing2006* 36 (1): 36–40.

  – Mean arterial pressure < 70 or > 130 mmHg
  – Heart rate < 45 or > 125
  – Respiratory rate < 10 or > 30
  – Complaints of chest pain
  – Change in mental status (lasting more than 10 minutes)

According to one study, 66% of patients had signs of instability for up to eight hours prior to the event.
Studies have shown that up to 70% of the calls to a Rapid Response Team were based on concerns
about the patient's respiratory status, accompanied by staff concern about a patient's deteriorating
condition.

Figure 9.1	*Critical thinking skills course—* *Additional resources handout (cont.)*

■ **"Brains in our Pocket" resources for nurses**

- PDA programs
    - See Audrey Snyder's chapter "PDA Use" in P. G. Zimmermann and R. D. Herr, 2006, *Triage Nursing Secrets* (St. Louis: Mosby/Elsevier) for suggested programs and sources to obtain them.

- Print:
    - Myers, E. 2003. *RNotes: Nurse's Clinical Pocket Guide.* Philadelphia: FA Davis.

■ **Good sources of test questions**

- LaCharity, L. A, C. D. Kumagai, and B. Bartz. 2005. *Prioritization, Delegation & Assignment Practice Exercises for Medical-Surgical Nursing.* St. Louis: Mosby/Elsevier.

- Springhouse. 2006. *NCLEX-RN: 250 New-Format Questions.* Philadelphia: Lippincott Williams & Wilkins.

- Rayfield, S., and L. Manning. 2004. *NCLEX-RN 101: How to Pass!,* 5th ed. Gulf Shores, AL: ICAN.

■ **Aids for writing better test questions**

- Bosher, S. 2003. "Linguistic bias in multiple-choice nursing exams." *Nursing Education Perspectives* 24 (1): 25–34.

- Zimmermann, P. G. 2005. "Writing effective test questions." *Journal of Emergency Nursing* 32 (1): 106–109.

■ **Concept mapping**

- Carpenito-Moyet, L. J. 2005. *Understanding the Nursing Process: Concept Mapping and Care Planning for Students.* Philadelphia: Lippincott Williams & Wilkins.

| Figure 9.1 | *Critical thinking skills course—Additional resources handout (cont.)* |

- Schuster, P. M. 2000. "Concept mapping: Reducing clinical care plan paperwork and increasing learning." *Nurse Educator* 25 (2): 76–81.

■ **Critical thinking books**

- Rubenfeld, M. G., and B. K. Scheffer. 2006. *Critical Thinking Tactics for Nurses.* Sudbury, MA: Jones and Bartlett.

- Lipe, S. K., and S. Beasley. 2004. *Critical Thinking in Nursing: A Cognitive Skills Workbook.* Philadelphia: Lippincott Williams & Wilkins.

■ **Generation X/multigeneration work force**

- Duchscher, J. E. B., and L. Cowin. 2004. "Multigenerational nurses in the workplace." *Journal of Nursing Administration* 34 (11): 493–501.

- Lower, J. 2006. *A Practical Guide to Managing the Multigenerational Workforce: Skills for Nurse Managers.* Marblehead, MA: HCPro.

- Raines, C. 2002. "Managing Generation X Employees" in P. G. Zimmermann's *Nursing Management Secrets.* Philadelphia: Hanley & Belfus.

- Raines, C. 1997. *Beyond Generation X.* Menlo Park, CA: Crisp.

- Sacks, P. 1996. *Generation X Goes to College.* Chicago and LaSalle, IL: Open Court.

■ **Example of a worst-case scenario**

- Zimmermann, P. G. (2003) "Lessons learned: On watching for zebras." *Journal of Emergency Nursing* 29 (1): 85–86.

| Figure 9.1 | Critical thinking skills course— Additional resources handout (cont.) |

■ Aids specific for triage/ED nursing

- Canadian Association of Emergency Physicians (CAEP). 1999. "Canadian emergency department triage and acuity scale implementation guidelines." *Journal of Canadian Association of Emergency Physicians* 1 (3): Supplement.

- Cohen, Shelley. 2002. *101 Triage Tips*. Hohenwald, TN: Health Resources Unlimited.

- Grossman, V. G. A. 2003. *Quick Reference to Triage*, 2nd ed. Philadelphia: Lippincott Williams & Wilkins.

- McNair, R. S. 2005. "It takes more than string to fly a kite: 5-Level acuity scales are effective, but education, clinical expertise, and compassion are still essential." *Journal of Emergency Nursing* 31 (6): 600–603.

- Terenzi, C. 2000. "The triage game." *Journal of Emergency Nursing* 26 (1): 66–69.

- Zimmermann, P. G., and R. D. Herr. 2006. *Triage Nursing Secrets*. St. Louis: Mosby/Elsevier.

- Zimmermann, P. G. 2003. "Tricks for the ED trade." *Journal of Emergency Nursing* 29 (5): 453–458.

- Zimmermann, P. G. 2002. "Triaging lower abdominal pain." *RN* 65 (12): 52–58.

Source: Polly Gerber Zimmermann, RN, MS, MBA, CEN

 Critical Thinking in the Emergency Department

| Figure
9.2 | *Unfolding teaching scenarios
for emergency nurses* |

(Note: Italics are directions for instructor or points to state/ask)

SCENARIO 1

A 27-year-old nursing student is brought to the emergency department because she fainted while watching a resident insert a central line. Students with her indicate there was no seizure activity nor head trauma. The nursing instructor with her stated she got an initial blood pressure of 70/40, 100. An IV was started on the unit with a bolus of 200cc, current blood pressure is 120/80.

What else do you want to know?

If the learner asks:	Respond with:
True loss of consciousness?	Yes, "everything went black"
Ate?	Yes, glucose was 88 mg
Other medical conditions?	Denies
Pregnant?	Denies, test negative
Alcohol, drugs?	Denies

How do you want to handle this?

What essential etiology do you need to rule out?

What essential piece of information do you want to ask?

Answer:
Any true loss of consciousness must have a cardiac etiology ruled out.

  • *Did you assume that cardiac couldn't be a factor because of her age?*

| *Figure* 9.2 | *Unfolding teaching scenarios for emergency nurses (cont.)* |

- *Did you assess the characteristics of her pulse (regular)?*

- *Did you assume it was just "nerves" because she is a nursing student? Would you have handled it differently if she had been an elderly woman at home?*

A key question to distinguish between dizziness/faint (feeling weak), vertigo (sense of movement, nystagmus), and syncope (true loss of consciousness) is, "What did you feel like right before this happened?"

Outcome of this actual case:
- She felt her heart pounding and racing, "I knew I was going to faint."

- Related it had happened twice before.

- Eventual outcome was a cardiac structural defect, exacerbated by her current anemia, stress, and fatigue (it was at the end of the year).

Lessons:
- Always use frequency of incidence to help "rule in" but not to rule out. Every rule has an exception. Were you less likely to think cardiac because of the patient's age and circumstances?

- Always rule out cardiac with true syncope (loss of consciousness)

SCENARIO 2*

A 46-year-old woman was in outpatient surgery to have a portacath insertion for chemotherapy for her pancreatic cancer. The conscious sedation procedure was done with benzodiapezine midazolam (Versed) and narcotic morphine, with oxygen being administered at 2 liters per nasal cannula. The patient became unresponsive and diaphoretic.

Figure

9.2

Unfolding teaching scenarios for emergency nurses (cont.)

Outpatient surgery staff performs the following actions:

- Vital signs: 100/60, 90, 16, pulse oximeter 96%: similar to baseline.
- Cardiac monitor showed normal sinus rhythm (NSR)
- Fluid bolus of 0.9 NS 200cc given with no response.

Patient is transferred to the emergency department. *What do you want to do?*

If someone immediately answers "glucose," do not respond. Others will give some of the other answers and respond to those.

If the learner asks:	Respond with:
Retake vital signs	Same
Airway	Nasal trumpet is inserted, oropharynx is suctioned and is clear
Glasgow Coma Scale (GCS)/neurological assessment?	GCS is 7, e.g., patient is in a "coma"
Administer benzodiazepine reversal agent flumazenil (Romazicon/Mazicon)	No response
Administer narcotic reversal agent naloxone hydrochloride (Narcan)	No response

Wait—this is when critical thinking takes place.

If no idea after 30 seconds, repeat again . . . a portacath for pancreatic cancer when she became unresponsive and **diaphoretic***.*

If no response, *"What other conditions cause sudden diaphoretic unresponsiveness?"*

Glucose, 35mg.

| Figure 9.2 | Unfolding teaching scenarios for emergency nurses (cont.) |

Outcome:

Responds to a half ampule of Dextrose 50%

Lessons:

- Glucose is always the "sixth vital sign" for sudden abrupt loss of consciousness
- Don't let the "red herring" pull you away from the basics

*Adapted from a true case in the Triage Decisions column. Molitor, L. 2002. "An unconscious diaphoretic 46-year-old woman." *Journal of Emergency Nursing* 28 (4): 367–368.

SCENARIO 3*

A 60-year-old man presents to triage complaining of back pain.

What is your initial impression? WAIT.

Muscular back pain is a "dime a dozen" in any emergency department.

What else do you want to know?

Figure

9.2

Unfolding teaching scenarios
for emergency nurses (cont.)

If the learner asks:	Respond with:
Vital signs	160/90, 96, 22
Allergies	None
Medications	ASA, antihypertensive
Medical history	Hypertension. No history of known injury or trauma Ask: *Does this strike you as unusual—no history of back pain, no causative history if this is typical muscular backache?*
Description of the pain	Gnawing, comes and goes, severe. Can't give it a number. *Nurse notes that the patient is rubbing his legs.*

What else do you want to do, know, or assess?

What potential lethal causes ("worst-case scenarios") do you want to ensure are not happening?

WAIT.

Nurse assessed his feet, pale with petechia noted.

Made emergent triage based on this significant finding.

Outcome:
Had a dissecting aneurysm, emergency surgery with good outcome.

| Figure 9.2 | Unfolding teaching scenarios for emergency nurses (cont.) |

Lessons:

- Go with your gut: If something seems unusual, it probably is.

- When you hear hoof beats, think horses not zebras. But there are some zebras out there.

- Atypical is typical in elderly.

- Can't diagnose in triage, but good assessment/history alerts nurse to the proper sense of urgency. Note his risk factors: HTN, age.

*Adapted from a true case in the Triage Decisions column. Moliter, L. 1999. "A 67-year-old man with back pain, pale feet, and hypertension." *Journal of Emergency Nursing* 25 (3): 246–247.

SCENARIO 4

A 60-year-old man presents by EMS to triage for a complaint of back pain. He is a janitor and the pain started after mopping the floor. Initial vital signs were 150/90, 88, 16, 20. Medical history is negative except for hypertension treated with an ACE inhibitor, and smokes a pack of cigarettes a day.

What else do you want to know?

If the learner asks:	Respond with:
Pain description (PQRST)	Sharp, comes and goes, midback, "7"; pain was relieved by the time the paramedics arrived.

What is your initial impression?
- Muscular pain

Classic findings for this common problem?
- Lower back (L4-5/S1 at highest risk due to bearing weight and structural weakness)

    Critical Thinking in the Emergency Department

Figure 9.2	*Unfolding teaching scenarios for emergency nurses (cont.)*

- Gradual onset over several hours?

- Does not radiate beyond knee

- Previous history?

- Disc protrusion

    What would help you to know if it was this?

    Ask:

    - Sudden onset? Recalls exact time of onset?

    - Radiates down the leg beyond the knee?

    - Maximum intensity at onset?

- Renal colic

    What would you ask/assess related to that?

    - Urine dipstick for blood

    - Previous history of renal colic?

- Caudal equine syndrome (central herniation of disc causing incontinence of bowel and bladder, inability to walk (versus pain with walking), or changes in neurological assessment

    What do you assess related to that?

    - Check legs bilaterally for strength and movement. Both 5+/5+.

    - Check bilateral pulses, finding right one is weaker. (Do not give this information if the learners do not ask for it).

While in triage, the pain becomes severe ("10," writhing), the patient become diaphoretic, and the pain is now described as moving into the lower back.

What are your thoughts now?

What else do you want to know and/or do besides telling the physician?

| Figure 9.2 | *Unfolding teaching scenarios for emergency nurses (cont.)* |

If the learner asks:	Respond with:
Description	"Ripping, tearing"

What cues you that this is no longer muscular pain?

- Sudden worsening (muscular pain is gradual in onset)
- Movement of the pain
- Systemic response
- Description of pain

If the learner mentions dissecting aneurysm, ask "What would you want to assess related to that possibility?"

- Blood pressure in both arms
- Bilateral pedal pulses
- "Blue toe syndrome"/foot petechiae from emboli

Outcome: Dissecting aneurysm, rushed to emergency surgery and recovered

Lessons learned:

- Always be sure to rule out the worst-case scenario occurring

- Sometimes patients "forget to read the textbook" and don't have the classic signs and symptoms, but the systemic involvement and sudden onset would alert the nurse to an emergent change

Source: Polly Gerber Zimmermann, RN, MS, MBA, CEN

Figure

9.3

Emergency department teachable moments

Case 1

A provider orders discharge for the patient that includes crutches for non–weight bearing of the right leg.

- The patient is 78 years old and lives alone. She has to climb stairs to access her bathroom and bedroom once home. During the crutch-walking demonstration it is obvious she does not have the coordination to handle the crutches and be non–weight bearing.

    ✓ Nurse recognizes unrealistic order for this patient

    ✓ Able to independently consider other options for this patient:
    - Walker
    - Reconsider non–weight bearing
    - In-home assistance
    - Family support for interim care elsewhere

    ✓ Collaboratively approaches provider with suggestions

    ✓ Successfully develops new nursing care plan for this discharge

Case 2

A burn patient is en route and you are orienting a new graduate nurse who is not assigned to this patient.

- Approach primary nurse prior to patient's arrival regarding role the nurse can play under your supervision

- Roles may include documentation, observation, initiating foley catheter, preparing IV lines, drawing and labeling lab for possible transfusion, etc.

<table>
<tr><td>*Figure*
9.3</td><td>*Emergency department teachable moments (cont.)*</td></tr>
</table>

✓   After the patient care is completed, meet with the new grad to discuss

- what priorities he or she noticed the nurses attended to, and why
- the role he or she played and how it felt being a part of this team
- what aspects he or she would have felt comfortable participating in without your observation
- what interventions on the part of the nurses required critical thinking
- what actions required knowledge of how to perform a task or procedure

Case 3

After receiving report from EMS regarding a patient they have received, the patient verbalizes physical complaints that do not match the EMS report.

• This is an opportunity to identify whether or not the nurse will "assume" EMS information is complete or correct.

✓   Does the nurse recognize the importance of the patient's perception?

✓   Does the nurse document the patient's statements in quotes?

✓   Does the nurse collaborate with EMS to verify other details?

Case 4

You're the preceptor for a new orientee who is working your assignment for the shift with you. As you check the crash carts in your area you notice items missing and some medications out of date.

✓   Can the nurse verbalize how noncompliance with restocking can affect care?

✓   Does the nurse know where and how to obtain the replacement items?

✓   Does the nurse know his or her responsibilities regarding any forms that need completion upon finding a crash cart that has not been properly restocked?

Figure 9.3	*Emergency department teachable moments (cont.)*

Case 5

Your orientee approaches you to share that yesterday the nurse she worked with had a patient with blunt trauma to the abdomen. The orientee was surprised that the nurse "spent so much time" trying to get an N/G tube down when the patient's blood pressure was dropping.

✓ Ask questions to reveal the critical thinking skills this nurse is or isn't using:

- What do you think the nurse should have been doing?

- Why do you think the blood pressure was dropping?

- Do you think the constant vomiting of blood had the potential to affect the airway?

- How would you approach a coworker who is helping you with your patient when you feel that his or her priorities are out of order?

Case 6

A nurse is caring for a diabetic patient who has received two liters of IV fluid for dehydration related to gastroenteritis. The patient is about to be discharged home. What actions should the nurse have taken prior to this and how should they have been documented?

✓ Ask questions that reveal the level of CTS the nurse is using:
- Is there a recent repeat blood sugar?
- Has the patient voided? How much?
- How does the patient feel?
- Does the patient know what signs to look for to alert him or her to return to the hospital?
- Has the patient been able to tolerate any po fluids prior to discharge?

Source: Shelley Cohen, RN, BS, CEN

Critical thinking skills and geriatric patients

Critical thinking requires knowledge, experience, and the ability to judge what is in the best interest of the patient.

- Be curious about things
- Ask pertinent questions
- Examine problems closely before assuming anything
- Seek resources and advice when you don't understand
- Reject advice that says, "That's the way we've always done it around here"
- Be open minded
- Identify incorrect information and reject it

1. **78-year-old male patient with a history of arthritis.**

   Patient states: "The medicine doesn't work. I don't feel any better."
   - What question will you respond to the patient with?
   - How can you clarify the patient's expectations of the medicine?
   - Is there really a medical problem, or is this an issue of lack of communication?

2. **67-year-old female patient with a history of hypertension presents with blood pressure of 176/112.**

   Patient states: "I feel just fine. I don't know what all the fuss is about."
   - What question will you respond to the patient with?
   - Can you clarify the patient's perception of what her diagnosis of hypertension means?
   - Do you need to verify her compliance with medical treatment since she claims to feel fine?

3. **92-year-old male has been examined by the provider. You are about to change his dressing and discharge him home.**

   Patient states: "The doctor just told me everything is okay. But I know something is wrong they are not telling me about." He is now crying and appears anxious.
   - What question will you respond to the patient with?
   - Other than his medical condition, what might his emotions be related to?

Source: Shelley Cohen, RN, BS, CEN

Figure

9.5

[Your facility] Critical Thinking Skills
[Date of program]

9:00–9:15	Introduction to critical thinking and course overview
9:15–10:00	Patient assessments
	Anatomy/physiology review
	Establishing the baseline
	Reassessments
10:00–10:15	Stretch break
10:15–11:30	Age-specific patients
	Include pediatric and/or geriatric specifics
	Geriatric
	Polypharmacy issues
	Atypical presentations
	Elder misuse and reporting
	Pediatric
	Social challenges
	Children as victims and reporting suspicion
	Medication specifics for children
11:30–12:15	Lunch
12:15–1:15	Red flags
	Patient statements/comments
	Family input
	Documentation specifics
	Case scenarios
1:15–1:30	Stretch break
1:30–2:30	Applying the knowledge
	When to call the doctor
	More case scenarios
2:30	Course evaluations

Source: Shelley Cohen, RN, BS, CEN

| Figure 9.6 | Instructor worksheet—Connecting words to spark critical thinking |

Following each of these patient statements, what question(s) should you consider?

(Instructor notes: What you want the nurse to consider.)

1. Patient states he or she has had no pain relief after the medication you gave him or her.

   (Instructor note: Why is there no pain relief?)

2. Blood pressure unchanged, remains systolic over 175.

   (Instructor note: Why is the systolic still high?)

3. Dressing change completed, wound appears unchanged from yesterday.

   (Instructor note: Did you expect the wound to look different today?)

4. The patient appears drowsier today.

   (Instructor note: Compared to what? Why is there a neurological change? What do the words "more drowsy" mean to the rest of the team?)

Figure 9.7	*Student worksheet—Connecting words to spark critical thinking*

Following each of these patient statements, what question(s) should you consider?

1. Patient states he or she has had no pain relief after the medication you gave him or her.

2. Blood pressure unchanged, remains systolic over 175.

3. Dressing change completed, wound appears unchanged from yesterday.

4. The patient appears drowsier today.

Figure

9.8

Worksheet—Relationship to critical thinking

How does each of these items below relate to critical thinking? Give one patient example for each.

Invasive therapy / treatment / indwelling devices

- Intravenous

- Catheters

- Tubes

    - Nasogastric

    - Suprapubic

    - Feeding

- Chest

- Colostomy

- Urostomy

- Dressings

- Wounds

- Orthopedic devices

     Critical Thinking in the Emergency Department

Figure	Worksheet—Vital signs
9.9	

In each set of adult vital signs below, what question would you ask the patient? What other areas would you assess?

Vital signs + Assessment = Critical thinking

"A critical thinker is able to reject information that is incorrect or irrelevant." —S. Ferrett

---

Case 1

Temp	97.4°F (rectal)
Pulse	118
Respirations	26
Blood pressure	128/72

Case 2

Temp	95.5°F (po)
Pulse	62
Respirations	30
Blood pressure	192/66

Case3

Temp	102.4°F
Pulse	78
Respirations	14
Blood pressure	78/52

<table>
<tr><td>Figure
9.10</td><td colspan="3">Worksheet—Red flag alerts</td></tr>
</table>

Patient statement/question	Makes you think . . .	Your response is . . .
That doesn't look like the pill I take at home.		
My dad has never been confused. He may be 94, but he is as sharp as a tack.		
I know you people think I'm nuts, but I am telling you: My daughter has never acted like this before.		
I think I am going to die. I feel like it is all over for me.		
I just don't feel right. I am not sure why.		
I didn't know I was having this done today.		
That's not what the other nurse told me to do.		
Do you know why that other nurse wouldn't give me anything for pain?		
My son left me this to eat, but I thought I wasn't supposed to have candy.		
My doctor told me yesterday I was having blood work done today. No one has been here to draw it.		
I heard on the TV last night that I shouldn't take this medicine any more. What do you think I should do?		
I am tired of being treated like a number. I want to go home! No one is telling me anything.		
Shouldn't I feel better by now?		

 Critical Thinking in the Emergency Department

Nursing education instructional guide

Target audience

- Chief nursing officers
- Directors of nursing
- Nurse managers
- Directors of education
- Staff development specialists
- VPs of nursing
- Nurse preceptors
- HR professionals

Statement of need

This practical guide to teaching and developing critical thinking includes strategies for designing and holding critical thinking courses, how to include critical thinking training in orientation, and how to encourage the ongoing development of critical thinking. Critical thinking skills help nurses become better decision makers and encourage independent practice. The book teaches nurse leaders, nurse managers, and staff educators how to develop critical thinking in the classroom and on the unit so they can incorporate critical thinking into everyday practice, both for novice nurses and ongoing development for advanced practitioners. (This activity is intended for individual use only.)

Educational objectives

Upon completion of this activity, participants should be able to

- describe the characteristics of the emergency department that require good critical-thinking skills

- identify the key aspects of critical thinking and how nurses develop competency

- analyze the factors that contribute to new graduates' lack of critical thinking and strategies to counteract this

- utilize the classroom environment to teach, promote, and support the development of critical thinking

- identify ways to incorporate critical thinking development into orientation programs and ways to evaluate nurses' progress

- discuss the role played by managers and educators in promoting environments that support critical thinking

- evaluate the challenges facing new and experienced nurses in incorporating critical thinking skills into practice and strategies to help meet expectations

- evaluate strategies to apply critical thinking to nursing documentation

Faculty

Shelley Cohen, RN, BS, CEN, is the founder and president of Health Resources Unlimited, a Tennessee-based healthcare education and consulting company *(www.hru.net)*. Through her seminars for nursing professionals, Cohen coaches and educates healthcare workers and leaders across the country to provide the very best in patient care. She frequently presents her work on leadership and triage at national conferences.

She has a background in emergency, critical care, and occupational medicine. Over the past 30 years, she has worked both as a staff nurse and nurse executive.

Polly Gerber Zimmermann, RN, MS, MBA, CEN, has been in active in emergency and medical-surgical nursing clinical practice for more than 29 years and involved in nurse educating for more than 10 years. She was the senior course manager for the nursing division of the National Center for Advanced Medical Education, and is a tenured assistant professor in the Department of Nursing at the Harry S. Truman College (Chicago). Under her guidance, the school's curriculum instituted an integration of prioritization principles and critical thinking that resulted in the school's students improving from below to above national average results in these areas on standardized test scores.

Accreditation/designation statement

This educational activity for three nursing contact hours is provided by HCPro, Inc. HCPro is accredited as a provider of continuing nursing education by the American Nurses Credentialing Center Commission on Accreditation.

Disclosure statements

HCPro, Inc. has a conflict-of-interest policy that requires course faculty to disclose any real or apparent commercial financial affiliations related to the content of their presentations/materials. It is not assumed that these financial interests or affiliations will have an adverse impact on faculty presentations; they are simply noted here to fully inform the participants.

Shelley Cohen and Polly Gerber Zimmermann have declared that they have no commercial/financial vested interest in this activity.

Instructions

In order to be eligible to receive your nursing contact hours for this activity, you are required to do the following:

1. Read the book *Critical Thinking in the Emergency Department: Skills to Assess, Analyze, and Act*
2. Complete the exam
3. Complete the evaluation

4. Provide your contact information on the exam and evaluation

5. Submit exam and evaluation to HCPro, Inc.

Please provide all of the information requested above and mail or fax your completed exam, program evaluation, and contact information to

Robin L. Flynn

Manager, Continuing Education

HCPro, Inc.

200 Hoods Lane

P.O. Box 1168

Marblehead, MA 01945

Fax: 781/639-0179

NOTE:

This book and associated exam are intended for individual use only. If you would like to provide this continuing education exam to other members of your nursing staff, please contact our customer service department at 877/727-1728 to place your order. The exam fee schedule is as follows:

Exam quantity	Fee
1	$ 0
2–25	$15 per person
26–50	$12 per person
51–100	$ 8 per person
101+	$ 5 per person

Continuing Education Exam

Name: _____

Title: _____

Facility name: _____

Address: _____

Address:_____

City: _____ State: _____ Zip: _____

Phone number: _____ Fax number: _____

E-mail: _____

Nursing license number: _____

(ANCC requires a unique identifier for each learner.)

Date completed: _____

1. **Which of the options below best completes the following sentence?**
    With rapidly changing multiple patient assignments and constant sorting, the ED nurse
    needs to have all the attributes of a critical thinker, and know how to use strategies that

    a. relax patients' families

    b. aid critical thinking

    c. inform physicians of the patient's status

    d. improve patients' conditions

2. **The most successful triage nurses are those who possess a combination of**

    a. experience and confidence

    b. several patients and multiple breaks

    c. critical thinking and experience

    d. patience and good interpersonal skills

3. **The ED nurse that recognizes the discharge orders from the provider are premature and the patient will need to wait for an evaluation by the mental health worker is**

   a. an independent thinker

   b. subject to a lawsuit for unlawful restraint

   c. not exploring consequences before making decisions or taking action

   d. acting beyond the scope of practice

4. **According to Benner, a nurse that views a situation as a whole rather than in parts and is able to develop a solution is**

   a. advanced beginner

   b. competent

   c. proficient

   d. technical

5. **According to Del Bueno's definition of critical thinking, which of the following is an essential aspect in a clinical setting:**

   a. The nurse thinks outside the box to create a novel nursing approach

   b. The nurse can state the five rights of all types of medication administration

   c. The nurse can define the meaning of ABCD prioritization

   d. The nurse does the right thing for the right reason

6. **A new graduate nurse that has little confidence in his or her skills and decision-making abilities has**

   a. unfamiliarity with the structure of the organization

   b. lack of clinical judgment

   c. lack of professional relationships

   d. lack of professional training

7. **To minimize the stress of new graduate nurses, consider**

   a. handing out stress balls during orientation

   b. suggesting they wait, assess, and hope for a solution

   c. using a mentor or assigning a buddy who builds a relationship and follows the nurse for at least one year

   d. avoiding support groups that introduce graduate nurses to the worries and stresses of their peers

 Critical Thinking in the Emergency Department

8. **True sudden beginning of symptoms can signal a catastrophic event. Which prioritization principle can this be applied to**

    a. trends

    b. systemic over local

    c. actual over potential

    d. onset

9. **To help new graduates identify worst-case scenarios,**

    a. give examples of actual cases and identify the worst-case complications

    b. have the new graduates witness worst-case scenarios

    c. discuss ethical consequences if worst-case scenarios are missed

    d. teach basic pathophysiology

10. **Aids to help create a classroom-learning environment include**

    a. use of a podium during presentations to communicate an air of expert authority

    b. avoiding the use of color, as it distracts the learner from paying attention to the speaker

    c. having a break every 90–120 minutes to avoid breaking the learners' concentration

    d. placement of posters around the classroom walls to promote learning even if the learners' eyes wander

11. **Which of the following would be most likely to help motivate a Generation X nurse learn?**

    a. Relate the material to a sense of duty to keep current

    b. Emphasize the role of authority of the expert instructor

    c. Play games as a method to teach the material

    d. Focus on the possibility of future promotions if learning is evident

12. **When new graduates are asked about their biggest fears and concerns about becoming professional nurses, they frequently mention**

    a. how to communicate with physicians

    b. they will be late for work

    c. they will feel left out and have trouble making friends at work

    d. they can't safely administer meds

13. Unfolding case scenarios provide information in staggered amounts, followed by

    a. outcomes

    b. results

    c. answers

    d. questions

14. In cooperative learning, the main advantage of a "think, pair, and share" exercise is that everyone

    a. participates

    b. has an opinion

    c. memorizes the objective

    d. develops a relationship

15. Which of the following is an effective way to use questions in a classroom setting?

    a. Ask trick questions

    b. Pose questions to stimulate thinking rather than yes/no questions

    c. Always let the most outspoken student answer

    d. Limit all questions to the end of class

16. When developing a self-assessment tool for new graduate nurses to measure their perception of their ability to perform at the critical thinking level, it is best to include items that reflect

    a. recall of information

    b. personality traits

    c. generic nursing skill

    d. history of the institution

17. As new nurses work through the orientation process, evaluating their ability to apply critical thinking in their clinical setting needs to be

    a. evidenced

    b. difficult

    c. strict

    d. general

18. Preceptors can help orientees develop and stimulate the use of critical thinking skills by

    a. minimizing emphasis on the ability to recognize when the skill or task is needed

    b. discouraging realistic time frames

    c. assuming the new hire understands the what, why, how, and when of delivering nursing care

    d. minimizing the emphasis on ability to perform skills and tasks

19. When nursing staff other than the preceptor are working with the orientee, it is _____ that the preceptor educates all staff on the importance of their roles, in assisting with the transition process of the newly hired nurse.

    a. not important

    b. essential

    c. somewhat important

    d. unnecessary

20. Managers and educators need to ensure a patient care environment that nurtures critical thinkers, stimulates them, and motivates them to engage in a discussion in their minds. This discussion is all about which of the following questions?

    a. Is this in the best interest of the organization?

    b. Is this in the best interest of myself?

    c. Is this in the best interest of the patient?

    d. Is this in the best interest of my learning process?

21. When considering how to improve the content of job descriptions, nurse managers should ask staff

    a. what they do on a regular basis that is not part of the job description

    b. to write a list of their favorite tasks

    c. to edit the job description

    d. nothing—nurse managers should not ask staff for assistance in improving the content of job descriptions

22. **A challenge that new graduate nurses face upon entering the workplace that directly affects their critical thinking abilities is**

   a. students have had too much clinical experience in school

   b. many nurses today enter a specialty straight out of school, rather than gaining years of experience first

   c. students have had so much clinical time that they have been exposed to too many challenging patients

   d. Students today do not have to contend with a shortage of nursing faculty

23. **To coach new graduate nurses through bad patient outcomes**

   a. do not allow them to have any grieving time through their error/omission

   b. even if the bad outcome was not related to something they did or did not do, allow a guilt trip to help them cope

   c. allow others to debrief the nurses before you do

   d. provide them with more than one opportunity to sit with a supportive mentor or preceptor to review the scenario that led to the patient outcome

24. **To encourage collaborative efforts between the medical staff and new graduate nurses**

   a. avoid introducing new graduates to too many members of the medical staff to avoid overwhelming the new graduates

   b. do not allow medical staff that has had previous negative experiences with new graduate nurses to interact with the new graduate nurses

   c. ask the medical staff to think back to their own internships and remind them that new graduates' critical thinking will develop with their support

   d. have new graduates in specialty areas stay out of practitioner offices

25. **Transforming critical thinking into the written format provides a legal record to support nurse's**

   a. patient outcomes related to any intervention

   b. right to work

   c. attendance

   d. ability to follow directions

Continuing education evaluation

Name: _____

Title: _____

Facility name: _____

Address: _____

Address: _____

City: _____ State: _____ Zip: _____

Phone number: _____ Fax number: _____

E-mail: _____

Nursing license number: _____

(ANCC requires a unique identifier for each learner.)

Date completed: _____

1. **This activity met the learning objectives stated:**

   Strongly agree   Agree   Disagree   Strongly disagree

2. **Objectives were related to the overall purpose/goal of the activity:**

   Strongly agree   Agree   Disagree   Strongly disagree

3. **This activity was related to my continuing education needs:**

   Strongly agree   Agree   Disagree   Strongly disagree

4. **The exam for the activity was an accurate test of the knowledge gained:**

   Strongly agree   Agree   Disagree   Strongly disagree

5. **The activity avoided commercial bias or influence:**

   Strongly agree   Agree   Disagree   Strongly disagree

6. **This activity met my expectations:**

   Strongly agree   Agree   Disagree   Strongly disagree

7. **Will this activity enhance your professional practice?**

    Yes   No

8. **The format was an appropriate method for delivery of the content for this activity:**

    Strongly agree   Agree   Disagree   Strongly disagree

9. **If you have any comments on this activity, please note them here:**

10. **How much time did it take for you to complete this activity?**

Thank you for completing this evaluation of our continuing education activity!

Return completed form to:

HCPro, Inc. • Attn: Robin L. Flynn • 200 Hoods Lane, Marblehead, MA 01945

Tel: 877/727-1728 • Fax 781/639-2982